The Complete Mediterranean Diet Cookbook

Quick and Easy Recipes That Help You Eat

Healthy and Stay in Shape
For Beginners and Advanced Users

Simon Kelley

TABLE OF CONTENTS

INTRODUCTION.. 6

THE MEDITERRANEAN DIET 9

THE PRINCIPLES OF THE DIET 14

THE BENEFITS 18

MINDSET FOR SUCCESS ON THE MEDITERRANEAN DIET 23

BREAKFAST 28

1. Sweet Potatoes with Coconut Flakes 28
2. Flaxseed & Banana Smoothie 28
3. Fruity Tofu Smoothie 28
4. French toast with Applesauce 29
5. Banana-Peanut Butter 'n Greens Smoothie 29
6. Baking Powder Biscuits 30
7. Oatmeal Banana Pancakes with Walnuts 30
8. Creamy Oats, Greens & Blueberry Smoothie 31
9. Banana & Cinnamon Oatmeal 31

LUNCH 32

10. Tomato and Halloumi Platter 32
11. Chickpeas and Millet Stew 32
12. Chicken Salad 33
13. Chicken Skillet 34
14. Tuna and Couscous 34
15. Chicken Stuffed Peppers 35
16. Turkey Fritters and Sauce 35
17. Stuffed Eggplants 36
18. Salmon Bowls 37

APPETIZERS 38

19. GREEK YOGURT (USED AS DIP) 38

20. LEMON GARLIC SESAME HUMMUS DIP 38   21. CREAMY GREEK YOGURT AND CUCUMBER 38

22. NACHOS 39

23. STUFFED CELERY 39   24. BUTTERNUT SQUASH FRIES 40

25. DRIED FIG TAPENADE 40

26. SPEEDY SWEET POTATO CHIPS 41

27. NACHOS WITH HUMMUS (MEDITERRANEAN INSPIRED) 41

28. PINEAPPLE MEDITERRANEAN DIP 41

29. MEDITERRANEAN INSPIRED TAPENADE 42

SALADS 43   30. LENTIL SALMON SALAD 43   31. PEPPY PEPPER TOMATO SALAD 43

32. BULGUR SALAD 44

33. TASTY TUNA SALAD 44

34. SWEET AND SOUR SPINACH SALAD 45

35. EASY EGGPLANT SALAD 45

36. SWEETEST SWEET POTATO SALAD 46

SOUPS & STEWS RECIPES 47

37. ITALIAN BROCCOLI & POTATO SOUP 47

38. BROCCOLI SOUP WITH GORGONZOLA 47

39. COMFORT FOOD SOUP 47

40. COMFY MEAL STEW 48

41. EXCITING CHICKPEAS SOUP 49

42. CLASSIC NAPOLI SAUCE 50

43. WINTER DINNER STEW 50

44. MEATLESS-MONDAY CHICKPEAS STEW 51

45. Fragrant Fish Stew 52

SIDES 53

46. Artichoke Hearts 53

47. Roasted Baby Potatoes 53

48. Scalloped Tomatoes 54   49.   Brussels   Sprouts   &   Pistachios 55   50.   Mashed   Celeriac 56

51. Fennel Wild Rice 56

52. Parmesan Broccoli 57

MEAT MAINS 59

53. Braised Beef In Oregano-tomato Sauce 59

54. Pork Chops and Herbed Tomato Sauce 59

55. Pita Chicken Burger with Spicy Yogurt 60

56. Beef Brisket and Veggies 60

57. Stewed Chicken Greek Style 61

58. Hot Pork Meatballs 62

59. Beef and Zucchini Skillet 62

SEAFOOD MAINS 64

60. Mussels with tomatoes & chili 64

61. Lemon Garlic Shrimp 64

62. Pepper Tilapia with Spinach 65

63. Spicy Shrimp Salad 65

64. Baked Cod in Parchment 66

65. Thai Tuna Bowl 66

66. Roasted Fish & New Potatoes 67

POULTRY MAINS ....
68

    67. TURKEY BURGERS WITH MANGO SALSA 68

    68. HERB-ROASTED TURKEY BREAST ....
    68

    69. CHICKEN SAUSAGE AND PEPPERS ....
    69   70.   CHICKEN   PICCATA 70

    71. ONE-PAN TUSCAN CHICKEN 70

    72. CHICKEN KAPAMA ....
    71

    73. SPINACH AND FETA–STUFFED CHICKEN BREASTS 72

VEGETABLES MAINS ....
74

    74. PEPPERS AND LENTILS SALAD 74

    75. OLIVES AND LENTILS SALAD 74

    76. LIME SPINACH AND CHICKPEAS SALAD 75

    77. BEANS AND CUCUMBER SALAD 75

    78. TOMATO AND AVOCADO SALAD ....
    76

    79. CORN AND TOMATO SALAD.. 76

    80. ORANGE AND CUCUMBER SALAD 77

    81. PARSLEY AND CORN SALAD 77

    82. LETTUCE AND ONIONS SALAD 78

    83. SWEET POTATO AND EGGPLANT MIX 78

    84. TOMATO AND BEANS SALAD 78

BEANS, RICE, AND GRAINS ....
80

    85. CHICKPEA AND RICE 80

    86. ONE-POT RICE AND CHICKEN 80

    87. GRAIN BOWL WITH LENTIL AND CHICKPEAS 81

    88. WHITE BEANS WITH VEGETABLES ....
    82

    89. GREEK WHEAT BERRY SALAD WITH FETA 83

    90. SKILLET BLACK-EYED PEASE AND SPINACH.. 84

    91. LENTIL SALAD WITH ORANGES 85

    92. BELL PEPPERS 'N TOMATO-CHICKPEA RICE 85

    93. SEAFOOD AND VEGGIE PASTA 86

    94. BREAKFAST SALAD FROM GRAINS AND FRUITS 86

PIZZA ....
88

95. Funghi & Aglio Pizza 88

96. Pizza Quattro Formaggi 88

97. Turkey Pepperoni Pizza... 89

98. Tuna & Rosemary Pizza 89

99. Tomato and Egg Breakfast Pizza 90

100. Easy Pizza Pockets 90

101. Mushroom-Pesto Baked Pizza 91

SNACKS & DRINKS 92

102. Garlic and Tomato Bruschetta 92

103. Crostini.. 92

104. Baby Shrimps 93

105. Spicy tomato to baked potatoes 94

106. Green beans with warm dressing and bacon 94

107. Rolls with lettuce 95

PASTA ....

97 108. Broccoli and Carrot Pasta Salad ....

97 109. Bean and Veggie Pasta ....

97

110. Roasted Ratatouille Pasta 98

111. Lentil and Mushroom Pasta... 99

112. Tomato Basil Pasta 99

DESSERT ....

101

113. Almond and Chocolate Butter Dip 101

114. Strawberry and Feta Delight 101

115. Simple Strawberry Yogurt Ice Cream 102

116. Pear with Honey Drizzles 103

117. Cherry and Olive Bites 103

118. Fluffed Up Chocolate Mousse 104

119. Chocolate Butter Dip 105

120. Mouthwatering Panna Cotta with Mixed Berry Compote 105

28 DAY MEAL PLAN ....

107

CONCLUSION ....

109

INTRODUCTION

Diet, also known as the Med Diet, is one of the best diets for your health Diet plays a significant role in your health and well-being. The Mediterranean

and longevity. The Mediterranean diet is known for being healthy and tasty. The Mediterranean diet is full of fresh vegetables, fruits, grains, and beans. You need to follow the Mediterranean Diet as closely as possible if you want to reap all the benefits.

The Mediterranean Diet is a diet that originated in the region of the Mediterranean Sea. It consists of a variety of plant-based foods, fish, olive oil, and wine. The diet is rich in fruits and vegetables and low in fat. The Complete Mediterranean Diet Cookbook is an excellent book for people who want to eat healthily. With over 250 recipes and 500+ food photos, this book is perfect for those who love to cook. What you consume is one of the most important things you can do for your health. "The Complete Mediterranean Diet Cookbook" best practices are built on the idea that eating the right foods can help us live longer, healthier lives.

The Mediterranean diet consists mainly of plant foods such as vegetables, fruits, beans, nuts, and whole grains. The Complete Mediterranean Diet Cookbook contains over 1,300 recipes with a focus on the Mediterranean diet. This book is full of healthy recipes, and it's easy to follow.

The Mediterranean diet is a diet based on foods and cooking traditions from the Mediterranean region. The Mediterranean diet has been the link to heart health and longevity, weight loss, reduced risk of chronic diseases, and better mental health. The Mediterranean diet is high in fiber, which helps promote satiety and healthy cholesterol levels. Much research shows that the Mediterranean Diet can lower heart disease rates, diabetes, and some cancers. While there are many ways to eat healthily, the Mediterranean diet is a great way to get the best nutrition. The Mediterranean diet emphasizes fruits, vegetables, whole grains, fish and poultry, and little red meat and sugar.

The Mediterranean Diet is a eating plan that has to lower the risk of many diseases, including heart disease. The Complete Mediterranean Diet Cookbook is a guide to eating for health and longevity. The book offers a variety of recipes for nearly every meal, with ingredients from the Mediterranean region. It's packed with recipes, but it also offers guidelines on implementing the diet into your own life.

There is a reason why the Mediterranean Diet is called the Med Diet.

The Med Diet is a lifestyle you live. It is a daily lifestyle, and it takes time. You have to make time.

The Mediterranean diet is a healthy and balanced diet rich in fiber, antioxidants, and phytochemicals. The Mediterranean Diet keeps the heart healthy and helps reduce the risk of heart attacks and strokes. The Mediterranean diet also lowers the risk of many diseases such as cancer and osteoporosis.

It is the best diet for health, weight loss, and longevity. The Mediterranean Diet is a highly-restrictive diet that consists of high-fiber foods like fruits, vegetables, nuts, and beans. The Complete Mediterranean Diet Cookbook by Sarah Ballantyne, a personal chef and one of the world's most influential food writers. The Complete Mediterranean Diet Cookbook is a resource that can help you create delicious, healthy recipes that can at any meal of the day. The cookbook with all sorts of recipes from breakfast to dinner and everything in between.

There is a reason why the Mediterranean Diet is called the Med Diet. The name of the diet invokes images of a seashore full of Mediterranean dishes. You can think about the hearts of the sea, mussels, and oysters lying on the sand, ready to be eaten.

However, there is nothing like this in real life, although the Mediterranean Diet includes fish and seafood. It also contains vegetables and fruits, which have a significant role in the Med Diet. The vegetarian dishes are also extremely diverse and in the Mediterranean Diet.

The Mediterranean Diet is simple. It is, in fact, straightforward. It is also a diet that can be followed by any style of life, as long as you live a lifestyle that is not too labor-intensive. Although it is not always possible to eat a Mediterranean Diet, the effects of doing so are undeniable. There is still something healthy about the Med Diet. Some nutritionists have been recommending the Med Diet for a long.

A lot of research and studies proving that the Mediterranean Diet effectively reduces heart ailments by either avoiding it entirely or reducing the damage done to it by the time it strikes.

Perhaps this is why it often comes as a surprise to people that something healthy is healthy about the Med Diet. They believe that dieting usually means that they have to stop eating everything and that they will have to stop eating one type of food or another. If they are vegetarians, they will need to find a route to adapt to the Med Diet.

There are families worldwide who are willing to change diet if followed by a lifestyle change, even if it is only for a brief time.

The Mediterranean Diet has a lot of benefits. It is an astonishing thing people have a lot of stress, or for the people who drink too much of a type of alcohol detrimental to their health. It is a good thing for people who want to lose weight. It is a good thing for people who want to prevent heart diseases.

It is a good thing for people who have an active life. The Mediterranean Diet can aid in the knowledge of trying something new. It can help keep the look of the skin glowing. It can help keep the joints limber.

THE MEDITERRANEAN DIET

T vitamins, minerals, antioxidants, and healthy fatty acids. However, the he healthy Mediterranean way of life is about eating balanced foods rich in Mediterranean diet is just one aspect of it. The Mediterranean way of life calls for regular physical exercise, plenty of rest, healthy social interaction, and fun. Balancing all these aspects was the secret of good health of the Mediterranean folk back in the day. However, only the Mediterranean diet is the primary focus of this book, and we will spend most of our time talking about just that.

Eat Healthy Fats

Remember: not all fats are created equal. Certain kinds of fats are beneficial, while others do more harm than good. Monosaturated fats and polyunsaturated omega-3 fatty acids, for example, are considered healthy. Omega-6 polyunsaturated fatty acids and saturated fats are unhealthy, and these harmful fats are primarily present in most typical food worldwide. The United States, for example, absolutely loves saturated fats. According to a survey, saturated fats constitute 11% of an average American's total calories, which is a very high number compared to an average Mediterranean resident, who consumes less than 8% of his/her calories through saturated fat. If you wish to switch to the healthy Mediterranean way of life, the first thing to do is change the oils you consume. Eliminating fats like butter and lard in favor of more nourishing oils like olive oil would be the place to start.

Consume Dairy in Moderation

We all love cheese. Dairy products are delicious, nutritious, and excellent sources of calcium and should be consumed in moderation if you're following the Mediterranean diet.

Consume Tons of Plant-Based Foods

As we saw in the pyramid, fruits, vegetables, legumes, and whole grains form the basis of the Mediterranean diet. So, it is a good idea to eat five to ten servings of these in a single day, depending on your appetite. Eat as much of these as you want, but don't overeat. Fresh, unprocessed plants are best, so always be on the lookout for the best sources of these around you!

Consume Seafood Weekly

As we've talked about before, one benefit of living close to the sea is the easy access to seafood. However, seafood holds a lower priority than plant-based foods in the Mediterranean diet and should d in moderation. If you're a vegetarian, consider taking fish oil supplements to get those omega-3 fatty acids into your system. Better yet, considering shunning your vegetarianism and eating seafood to get the vital nourishment only seafood can provide.

Consume Meat Monthly

Red meat used to be a luxury for the Mediterranean people back in the day. Although not completely off-limits, you should try and reduce your red-meat intake as much as possible. If you love red meat, consider consuming it no more than two times per month. And even when you eat it, make sure the serving size of the dish's essence is small (two to three-ounce serving). The main reason to limit meat intake is to limit unhealthy fats going into your system. As we talked about before, saturated fats and omega-6 fatty acids are not suitable for health, but unfortunately, red meat contains significant quantities. As a beef lover myself, I eat a two-ounce serving of it per month, and when I do eat it, I make sure there are lots of vegetables on the side to satiate my hunger.

Drink Wine!

Love wine? Well, it is your lucky day. A glass of wine is a common practice in the Mediterranean regions. Red wine is perfect for the heart, and it is an excellent idea to consume a glass of red wine twice a week. Excess of everything is terrible, and wine is no exception, so keep it in check. If you're already suffering from health conditions, it is a good idea to check with your doctor before introducing wine to your daily diet.

Work Your Body

Now you don't have to hit the gym like a maniac to work your body. Walking to your destination instead of driving, taking the stairs instead of the lift, or kneading your dough can all get the job done. So, be creative and work your body when you can. Better yet, play a sport or just hit the gym like a maniac. As I said at the start, you don't have to have to, but it will.

Enjoy a Big Lunch

Lunch was usually the meal of the day when the Mediterranean residents sat with their families and took their time enjoying a big meal. It strengthens social bonds and relaxes the mind during the most stressful time of the day when you're just halfway done with your work probably.

Have Fun with Friends and Family

Spending a few minutes per day doing something fun with your loved ones is great for de-stressing. Today, we don't understand the importance of this, and people feel lonely, and in some cases, even depressed. Just doing this one thing has the power to solve a huge chunk of the problems our modern society faces.

Be Passionate

The Mediterranean people are passionate folk. Living on or close to sun-kissed coasts, their passion for life is naturally high. Being passionate about something in life can take you a long way towards health and wellness.

Benefits of the Mediterranean Diet

Now that we have talked about how you can follow the Mediterranean lifestyle, we should speak in detail about all the benefits you will get to reap if you are successful.

The Diet Fights Free Radicals

In today's world, we have high exposure to harmful elements like vehicle exhaust, industrial waste, water contaminants, toxic foods, etc. These cause the free radicals in the body to escalate, increasing the risk of chronic diseases of the heart or even fatal diseases like cancer! Hence, it is vital to keep these free radicals in check as much as possible. The best way of doing so naturally is to eat a diet rich in antioxidants, like the Mediterranean diet.

The Diet is Rich in Phytochemicals

We know that plants are rich in vitamins and minerals, but few know that they with chemicals called phytochemicals. These are healthy chemicals in plants that provide numerous health benefits to the body, promote heart health, and help prevent certain cancers. Ever wondered why different fruits and vegetables exhibit different colors? The reason is the presence of various phytochemicals. Hence, it is possible to tell what kind of phytochemical a plant-based food merely contains by looking at its color. Refer to the table below to gain some phytochemical knowledge.

The Diet is Rich in Vitamin D

The human body gets vitamin D from food sources and exposure to sunlight. The Mediterranean residents have access to both and hence have good vitamin D. Some attribute their good health to their high vitamin D levels and right reason. Scientific research has demonstrated the numerous health benefits of the vitamin, and a few of these are listed below:

- Guards against Osteoporosis
- Reduces the risk of certain cancers
- Reduces the risk of coronary artery disease
- Reduces vulnerability to common infections such as the common flu

More Healthy Fats in Your Diet has multiple health benefits that include:

- •A lower risk of heart disease
- •Enhanced insulin function and blood sugar control

- Lower cholesterol levels
- Reduced inflammation in the body
- Body weight management
- Enhanced immune system function
- Management of behavioral issues

More Fiber in Your Diet

It is common knowledge that fiber is excellent for health. The best sources of fiber are fruits, vegetables, whole grains, and legumes. All of these ingredients are dominant in the Mediterranean diet, and hence by following the Mediterranean diet, you can quickly achieve your daily fiber goals. Fiber has multiple benefits for the body, a few of which are listed below:

- Helps maintain a healthy gastrointestinal tract by reducing constipation
- Decreases total cholesterol and harmful cholesterol levels, hence promoting heart health
- Reduces the rate at which sugar is absorbed into the bloodstream, therefore helping maintain healthy blood sugar levels
- Since the body can't break down fiber for energy, it effectively has zero calories but still fills up the stomach, hence reducing your calorie intake

More Functional Foods in Your Diet

Some foods provide specific health benefits other than primary nutritional benefits. These foods are called functional foods, and they are quite common in the Mediterranean diet. The table below shows the best available foods to always have in your pantry, along with the benefits they provide.

Food Benefits

Extra-virgin olive oil: Extra-virgin olive oil is loaded with monounsaturated fats and is an excellent source of phytochemicals, including polyphenolic compounds, squalene, and alpha-tocopherol. Health benefits include cardiovascular health, cancer prevention/protection, and immune-boosting.

Lemons (zest and juice) - Citrus bioflavonoids benefit both cholesterol and triglycerides. Lemon is also a dense source of vitamin C and exhibits antiinflammatory properties.

THE PRINCIPLES OF THE DIET

Look for Short Ingredient List: The bulk of the food is listed according to Learn How to Understand Nutrition Labels weight and is usually the first ingredient. If you don't recognize an element, place it back on the shelf! Consider using products that have no more than five ingredients. The longer ingredients probably are the result of unnecessary extras, including artificial preservatives.

Check Serving Sizes: Packages often time contain more than a single serving. Visualize how many calories and the amount of sugar is in a single container. Thus, you need to check the serving size first.

Discover Calorie Counts: It is essential to check the labels' calorie count since they are significant during your Mediterranean diet plan.

Check the Percent of Daily Value: The daily value will tell you how many nutrients are in each serving of a packaged item.

Get More Of These Nutrients: Look for calcium, iron, fiber, vitamin A, and vitamin C.

The Label Explained d

- Serving Information at the Top: This provides the size of one serving and per container.
- Check the total calories per serving and container.
- Limit certain nutrients from your diet.
- Provide yourself with plenty of beneficial nutrients
- Understand the % of daily value section.
- Avoid These Foods
- Processed Meat Products: Hot dogs, processed sausages, bacon

You will still need to pay attention when purchasing olive oil because it may have been extracted from the olives using chemicals or possibly diluted with other cheaper oils, such as canola and soybean. You need to be aware of refined or light olive or regular oils. The Mediterranean diet plan calls for the use of extra-virgin olive oil because it has been standardized for purity using natural methods providing the sensory qualities of its excellent taste and smell. The oil is high in phenolic antioxidants, which makes—real—olive oil beneficial.

Beverage Options: Maintaining a healthy body requires plenty of water, and the Mediterranean diet plan is not any different. Tea and coffee are allowed, but you should avoid fruit juices or sugar-sweetened beverages that contain large amounts of sugar.

White Meats: White meats are high in minerals, protein, and vitamins, but you should remove any visible fat and the skin.

Potatoes: It would be best if you considered that they contain large amounts of starch, leading to glucose, which can be harmful and place you at risk of type 2 diabetes.

Sweets and Desserts: Bread, cakes, and desserts should result in small quantities, as a special treat. Not only is sugar a temptation for type 2 diabetes, but it can also develop tooth discoloration. Many times, they may also include more significant levels of saturated fats. You can receive some nutritional value, but as a general rule—stick to small portions.

Improve the Flavor of Foods

Her herbs and spices provide additional flavor and aroma to your foods while on the diet plan. It will also help reduce the need for salt or fat while you're preparing your meals. Spices and herbs that adhere to a traditional Mediterranean Diet's standards include chills, lavender, tarragon, savory, sumac, and avatar.

These are a few more ways you can benefit from spices and herbs:

Anise Benefits: You can improve digestion as well as help reduce nausea and alleviate cramps. Prepare some anise tea after a meal to help treat indigestion and bloating gas as well as constipation.

Bay Leaf Benefits: Bay leaves contain magnesium, calcium, potassium, and Vitamins A & C. You are promoting your general health, and it is also proven to be useful in the treatment of migraines.

Basil Benefits: You can receive aid in digestion, help with gastric diseases, and help reduce flatulence. You can also protect your heart health, help reduce stress and anxiety, and help manage your diabetes. The next time you have dandruff issues, try rubbing them in your scalp after shampooing. The chemicals help eliminate dandruff and dry skin.

Black Pepper Benefits: Pepper promotes nutrient absorption in the tissues all over your body, speeds up your metabolism, and improves digestion. The main ingredient of pepper is a pipeline, which gives it a spicy taste. It can boost fat metabolism by as much as 8% for up to several hours after. As you will see, it throughout your healthy Mediterranean recipes.

Cayenne Pepper Benefits: The secret ingredient in cayenne is capsaicin, a natural compound that gives the peppers fiery heat. It provides a sharp increase in your metabolism. The peppers are also rich in vitamins, useful as an appetite controller, smoothest out digestion issues, and benefit your heart health.

Sweet & Spicy Cloves Benefits: Add cloves to hot tea for a spicy flavor. The antiseptic and germicidal ingredients in cloves will help with many types of pain, including the relief of arthritis pain, gum and tooth pain, aids in digestive problems, and helps to fight infections. Use the clove oil as an antiseptic to kill bacteria in fungal infections, itchy rashes, bruises, or burns. Just the smell of cloves can help encourage mental creativity.

Ground Chia Seeds Benefits: The seeds can absorb up to 11 times their weight in liquid. Be sure to add plenty of water and soak them for at least 5 minutes before using them in your recipes. Otherwise, you will have some uncomfortable digestion after eating them. Be sure to remain hydrated.

Cumin Benefits: The flavor of cumin has as spicy, earthy, nutty, and warm. It's as traditional medicine. It can help promote digestion and reduce foodborne infections. It is also beneficial for promoting weight loss and improving cholesterol and blood sugar control.

Fennel Benefits: You can receive potassium, sodium, vitamin A, calcium, vitamin C, iron, vitamin B6, and magnesium from fennel. Your bone health will show improvement with phosphate and calcium, which are excellent for your bone structure—iron and zinc or crucial for collagen production. Your heart health with vitamin C, folate, potassium, and fiber provided in fennel.

Garlic Benefits: Garlic leads the charge on lowering your blood sugar and assisting you in weight loss. It helps control your appetite.

Ginger Benefits: Ginger is an effective diuretic that increases urine elimination. It is also known for its cholesterol-fighting properties as a metabolism and mobility booster. Ginger also helps fight bloating issues.

Marjoram Benefits: This is used in the diet to promote healthy digestion, assist in the management of type 2 diabetes, helps to rectify hormonal imbalances, and also helps promote restful sleep and a sound mind.

Mint Benefits: can be use mint for the treatment of nasal congestion, nausea, dizziness, and headaches. It helps to improve blood circulation, improves dental health, and helps colic in infants. Mint helps to prevent dandruff and pesky head lice.

Oregano Benefits: Oregano is very easily added to your diet and is rich in antioxidants, and may also help fight bacteria. Oregano is also suitable for treating the common cold since it helps reduce infections, helps kill off intestinal parasites, and is also beneficial in treating menstrual cramps. One huge plus is that it also supports the body with nutrients to help support weight loss and improve digestion.

Parsley Benefits: You can help your skin, prostate, and digestive tract by making use of its high levels of a flavonoid called aligning. It contains a powerful antioxidant and inflammatory power as well as providing remarkable anti-cancer properties.

Rosemary Benefits: The spice is known to increase hair growth, may help relieve pain, eases stress, and also helps reduce joint inflammation.

THE BENEFITS

What are the Benefits of a Mediterranean Diet?

Where will go over just a few of the many improvements you can experience with your health when you start the Mediterranean diet.

Heart Health and Reduced Risk of Stroke

They maintained healthy blood pressure, blood sugar and staying within a healthy weight, resulting in optimal heart health. Your diet directly affects each of these components—those who are at greater risk to begin adhering to a low-fat diet. A low-fat diet cuts out all fats, including those from oils, nuts, and red meats.

The Mediterranean diet also stresses the importance of daily activity and stress reduction by enjoying quality time with friends and family. Each of these elements, along with eating more plant-based foods, significantly improves heart health and reduces the risk of many heart-related conditions. By increasing your intake of fresh fruits and vegetables while adding in regular daily activities, you improve not just your heart health but overall health.

Reduces Age-Related Muscle and Bone Weakness

Eating a well-balanced diet that provides you with a wide range of vitamins and minerals is essential for reducing muscle weakness and bone degradation. It is imperative as you age. Accident related injuries such as tripping, falling or slipping while walking can cause severe damage. As you age, this becomes even more of a concern as some simple falls can be fatal. Many accidents occur because of weakening muscle mass and the loss of bone density. Women, especially those entering the menopause phase of their life, are at a greater risk of serious injury from accidental falls because the estrogen levels decline significantly—this decrease in estrogen results in a loss of bone and muscle mass. The reduction of estrogen can also cause bone-thinning, which over time develops into osteoporosis.

Maintaining healthy bone mass and muscle agility as you age can be challenging. When you are not getting the proper nutrients to promote healthy bones and muscles, you increase your risk of developing osteoporosis. The Mediterranean diet offers you a simple way to fulfill the dietary needs necessary to improve bone and muscle functioning.

Plant-based foods, unsaturated fats, and whole grains help provide you with the necessary balance of nutrients that keep your bones and muscles healthy. Sticking with a Mediterranean diet can improve and reduce the loss of bone mass as you age.

Reduces the Risk of Alzheimer's

Alzheimer's disease is a significant cognitive decline. Those with Alzheimer's suffer from:

- Disorientation
- Memory Loss
- Inability to think clearly
- Speech problems
- Impaired judgment
- Visual and spatial disorientation

Alzheimer's is a common brain disorder in older adults, 60 years of age or older, but the first signs of Alzheimer's can be present in adults as young as 30. The condition can progress fast or slowly, depending on how quickly the brain's neurons begin to die off. Though the decline starts in the hippocampus area of the brain, it becomes widespread as it progresses.

Individuals with Alzheimer's show a significant increase in beta-amyloid proteins in the brain and have a much lower level of brain energy. None of the participants showed signs of dementia, and 34 of them adhered to a Mediterranean diet while 36 followed a standard Western diet. The scans showed that those on the Western diet had significant loss in brain energy levels and increased beta-amyloid build-up instead of those on the Mediterranean diet (Mediterranean Diet May Slow Development, 2018). The study highlights how simple lifestyle changes, such as those suggested on the Mediterranean diet, can help reduce the risk of Alzheimer's and other cognitive declines.

It indicates that diet can impact the leading two signifiers of the development of Alzheimer's disease. Just as diet can impact other areas of your health, it can affect your brain health as well. Cholesterol, blood sugar, and blood vessel health can contribute to your risk of developing Alzheimer's disease. The most common fuel sources for the brain are fresh fruits, which supply vital vitamins and nutrients. When processed foods, refined grains, and added sugars too often, it impairs the brain's functionality as these foods release toxins into the body. These toxins then cause widespread inflammation, and the brain begins to build up plaque, which causes a malfunction to cognitive ability (Nutrition and Dementia, 2019).

The Western diet consists of several foods that increase the risk of Alzheimer's disease, such as processed meat, refined grains like white bread and pasta, and added sugar. Foods that contain diacetyl, which is a chemical commonly used in the refinement process, increase beta-amyloid plaque build-up in the brain. Microwaveable popcorn, margarine, and butter are some of the most consumed foods that contain this harmful chemical. It is no wonder that Alzheimer's is becoming one of the leading causes of death among Americans.

On the other hand, the Mediterranean diet includes a wide range of foods that boost memory and slow down cognitive decline. Dark leafy vegetables, fresh berries, extra virgin olive oil, and fresh fish contain brain-boosting vitamins and minerals that can improve brain health. The Mediterranean diet can help you make the necessary diet and lifestyle changes that significantly decrease your risk of Alzheimer's.

Reduces Risk of Parkinson's disease

Parkinson's condition is a slowly improving neurodegenerative sickness that affects the dopamine-producing neurons in the brain. Those with Parkinson's disease will suffer from:

- Tremors
- Muscle stiffness
- Balance troubles
- Difficulty walking
- Depression
- Sleep problems
- Cognitive disruptions

Genetics and environmental factors have to understand better what causes one to develop Parkinson's disease. While genetics plays a factor in exposure to pesticides, herbicides, high cholesterol, low vitamin D levels, and limited physical activity can all increase the risk of Parkinson's disease.

Parkinson's disease is also common among individuals who have a higher level of oxidative stress. This damages the cell is the brain and can result in severe cognitive and physical decline. Antioxidants help reduce the risk of developing Parkinson's disease and help repair damaged cells and form stronger brain connections.

The Mediterranean diet encourages the consumption of antioxidant-rich foods such as fresh fruits and vegetables. Eating organic and locally grown fruits and vegetables reduces the risk of toxin exposure from pesticides and herbicides.

Those with Parkinson's are often encouraged to change their diet to include more healthy fats, like extra virgin olive oil, seeds, nuts, fresh fruits, organic vegetables, and whole grains. This diet recommendation is the basis of the Mediterranean diet. Individuals are also encouraged to reduce salt, sugar, and empty calorie foods, which the Mediterranean diet encourages.

Protects Against Type 2 Diabetes

Type 2 diabetes develops when your body can no longer produce or use the insulin produced properly. It causes blood sugar levels to spike to dangerous levels. Your blood sugar or glucose is what gives your body energy. It supplies fuel to your muscles, tissues, and cells so that they can function correctly. When glucose into the bloodstream, it signals the pancreas to begin to produce insulin so that the cells in the body can adequately absorb the glucose. Therefore, your cells cannot absorb enough of it, or the insulin is not correctly, so glucose is remaining in the body. A build-up of glucose in your body can cause a long list of health complications. The body may turn to use its muscle and fat to get the energy it needs. Blood vessels can also become damaged, which increases the risk of heart attack and stroke.

Those who are at the most significant risk of developing Type 2 diabetes include:

- Individuals who are overweight or obese
- Individuals who have a family history of Type 2 diabetes
- Individuals who have insulin resistance

The most common symptoms of Type 2 diabetes include

- Excessive fatigue
- frequent numbness of the hands or feet
- Tingling feelings in the hands and feet
- Regular headaches
- Vision difficulties
- Increase in urination
- Unquenchable thirst

Many individuals are unaware of their condition until a severe health complication arises because of the situation. Those with Type 2 diabetes are at a greater risk of heart attack, stroke, organ damage, loss of vision, hearing loss, and many other health conditions that can decrease quality of life and shorten your life-span.

What you eat contributes to insulin production and how efficiently your body can utilize the insulin produced. Carbohydrates specifically are converted to glucose for the body to use as energy. Many individuals eat too many unhealthy carbs, causing the body to be thrown out of balance and blood sugar levels to rise and remain elevated. The most common foods known to spike glucose levels are white bread, pasta, and sugary beverages. The excessive sugar and simple carbs found in these items cause the body to suddenly increase glucose, which the body often cannot handle fast enough.

MINDSET FOR SUCCESS ON THE MEDITERRANEAN DIET

12 Tips for Success

If you're motivated at this point to begin the Mediterranean diet and see the results for yourself, we are here to give you tips for success! The more informed you are about what to expect and what changes to make, the more success you will see as you adjust your life to this new diet.

Let's get started!

1.   Start using the right fats. For the Mediterranean diet, you need to switch to healthy oil like extra virgin olive oil. This oil is high in anti-inflammatory properties, which help the body. It means making the switch in your diet and removing unhealthy fats such as canola oil, vegetable oil, margarine, or butter. Olive oil should be your go-to for all your cooking needs. Avocado oil is a good substitute as well to keep on hand. Remind yourself that "less is more," and focus on minimizing your oil quantity but concentrate on its nutritional qualities.

2.   Get rid of what you can't eat. Like any diet, there will be an exact list of what you cannot eat - and the Mediterranean diet is no different. You want to get rid of those items to ensure you. That means getting rid of the unhealthy oils, processed foods and meats, sugary snacks and juices, fast food, and junk food. Get used to having fresh ingredients on hand and allowing yourself to meal plan and prep so you have a delicious meal waiting for you. If you had a favorite dish, you enjoyed, like lamb chops or fried chicken, see if you can find a Mediterranean diet alternative that is healthier for you.

3.   Get used to seafood. Your primary source of protein on the Mediterranean diet will be fish and seafood. If you're already a seafood lover, this is a great time to incorporate it more into your week where you would have eaten red meat. Remember, seafood is more than just fish - there's clams, shrimp, crab, lobsters, and so many other choices!. The more variety you incorporate into your diet, the more you will explore new recipes and find favorites.

4.   Try other sources of protein instead of red meat. If you often had red meat throughout the week, it can be tough adjusting to other protein sources. But it's a necessary switch and one you have to stick to, especially if you're hoping to fight symptoms of cardiovascular heart disease. Ease back on the red meat you include in your diet, so you have it only sparingly. Get used to fish, seafood, chicken, beans, and legumes as a source of protein. These are low in carbs and much healthier for you. Keep the meat as your "cheat meal," if you wish!

5.   Make vegetables the star of your meals. You want to have various vegetables on hand to incorporate it into your meals, or even as the main dish! Whether it's a healthy salad full of many vegetables, or a sautéed side of veggies with fish, you must include veggies in your meals as often as you can. Fiber, vitamins, and

minerals, which keeps us full in between meals, are primarily sourced through vegetables. It also ensures that your blood sugar levels stay stable. The Mediterranean diet is all about choosing plant-based ingredients, so you should experiment with more veggies and different ways to eat them.

6.   High sodium intake can cause health concerns and increase the risk of heart disease. Most of us are consuming too much salt and don't even realize it! Since the Mediterranean diet is all about heart health, try and experiment with various spices or herbs to add flavor to your meals rather than salt. It's great to experiment with different ethnic spices and see how what kind of taste it packs in your protein.

7.   You can choose to have wine but remember the limits you should follow. Some people love the red wine aspect of the Mediterranean diet, but it's important to remember that moderation is the key. Remember, this is only for red wine, and you cannot substitute other varieties of alcohol or hard liquor. If you're not a drinker, research suggests you could even potentially get the same health benefits by snacking on grapes! Some of the same heart-healthy properties of red wine in grapes. So, drinking is not necessary if you have health concerns or abstains from religious reasons.

8.   Make fruit your choice of dessert. We are used to thinking of dessert as something like cake or chocolate that we don't realize its effect on our health. Whether it's ripe melons, juicy orange slices, or sweet pears, these fruits and the natural sugars they contain are much better for your health and blood sugar levels than refined or artificial sugar. Get used to having fresh fruit on hand and treating it like the dessert platter in your house. It's delicious and healthy!

9.   Get moving! We've repeated over and over that the Mediterranean diet is not only a diet - it's a lifestyle change. To truly gain the Mediterranean people's benefits, you should try and incorporate physical activity into your routine. If you don't like a gym atmosphere, that means making voluntary choices to be more active in your day like walking, biking, swimming, hiking, performing more housework or chores around the house, etc. Whatever activity you prefer, get moving, and gain the health benefits that exercise offers!

10.   Plan your meals. As we mentioned before, excessive snacking can be your downfall when it comes to any diet! Even though the Mediterranean does encourage healthy snacking, the more calories you consume, the harder it will lose weight. It's more important to have a filling and healthy meal that will tide you over until the next mealtime! To do this, planning your meals is a great way to ensure your success. It allows you to plan, grocery shop, and prep your meals for the week. It reduces the temptation to grab fast food or go for something unhealthy because you know you have a meal waiting for you. Maybe use a day on the weekend to cut your veggies, marinate your fish fillets, and prepare some beans or lentils, so you have them for a couple of days in advance. It helps reduce food waste and keeps you motivated to eat what you've prepared!

11.   Try and share your mealtimes with people when you can. Another wonderful thing about the Mediterranean region is their cultural tradition of eating meals

together. It seems more common in the West to have quick "grab and go" meals alone at work or even at home. Everyone is a different schedule, and people eat when it's most convenient for them. Research has shown that sharing a meal can improve your mood, decrease stress levels, and even control the portion size of how much you're eating! It isn't possible with every meal every time, but it's excellent advice to encourage you to enjoy your food and mealtimes. So, next time, invite a colleague to eat lunch with you or invite a friend or family member over for dinner. They'll get to have a delicious meal, and you'll get to enjoy their company!

12.   be flexible and embrace the possibilities! The Mediterranean diet appeals to so many because of the flexibility it gives. You don't have to count calories, count macronutrients, or drastically cut the portions of your meals. You can eat so many varieties of foods, from fish, legumes, beans, vegetables, fruit, whole grains, poultry, dairy, and seafood. It gives you such variety in your meals to experiment with new recipes and new cuisines. Don't allow yourself to get bored when there are so many options available and new combinations you can try. Exercise is essential.

Your weight will depend on the amount of energy your body burns and how much energy you consume from beverage and food products. Before we begin, let's discuss a little about the science of how weight loss works. In short, if you consume more calories (more food) than your body can use, you add on the pounds. The excess or extra energy is converted to fat and in your body. If the number of calories you ingest equals the amount your body is using, your weight will remain stable or unchanged.

It requires your body to 'tap into' the stored body fat to obtain the additional energy needed. In one pound of fat, you receive about 3,500 calories. If you lower the calories by eating better on the plan, you can cut the calories by about 500 calories daily, resulting in one pound of weight loss weekly.

It is the beauty of the Mediterranean way of eating healthier; you don't want to drop the pounds too quickly, but you could with a new eating pattern. If you lose more than one kilogram or about 2.2 pounds, you might be losing muscle tissue instead of losing the unwanted fat. In short, that's why you need to get more exercise and eat fewer calories.

How to Proceed

It is crucial to increase your physical activities for about thirty minutes each day as part of your new diet regimen. You can begin slowly with a walk, go for a swim, go for a bicycle ride, or go for a jog.

If you have any other risk factors, such as smoking, maybe it is time to consider breaking the habit. Have your blood pressure frequently checked, so you know your diet plan is working for you.

Research has shown if you have a strict Mediterranean diet and exercise regularly, you can keep your weight under control. With the filling menus you will be planning, you won't be hungry and end up with unwanted calories or inches around your waistline. After all, a sedentary lifestyle is a major contributing factor to obesity.

Begin & Maintain a Regular Exercise Program

It would be best if you considered exercising 30-60 minutes daily as an integral part of healthy living choices. Regular physical activity benefits your strength, mood, and balance. If you've been living a more sedentary lifestyle, you need to speak with your doctor about a safe exercise regimen. Make sure you start slow. Progressively pick up the pace and regularity of your workouts.

Physicians suggest patients suffering from pressure issues should engage in dynamic, moderate-intensity aerobic exercise for a minimum of 1/2 hour each day. You can enjoy jogging, walking, swimming, or cycling five days each week. Start using a pedometer and set a new goal of activity using a base of 10,000 steps daily. Get started with a group of friends and walk or start a workout group.

Plan Walking With the Family. Start making Saturday morning your 'walk day' for the entire family. Take a Sunday walk instead of taking a Sunday drive. Walk instead of driving whenever you can. After the evening meal, go for a walk with the family. Make it a daily habit.

Go out Of Your Way to Walk:

If you take a bus, make an early stop, and walk part of the way.

When you go shopping, park a few aisles further away, and take a walk.

While you are window shopping, go for a brisk walk in the mall. If you have a choice of an elevator or the stairs, burn a few calories!

These are a few examples of how to burn those extra calories moderately:

- Housework - 60 min.
- Cycling - 6 min.
- Walking - 15 min.
- Running - 10 min.
- Swimming laps - 20 min.

Regular exercise can help strengthen your muscles and keep them flexible. One huge benefit is its ability to help improve your sense of well-being and control your weight. However, cardiac patients should avoid running and white training without getting professional advice.

Try a few of these moves:

When you reach a goal, the important thing is to reward yourself.

Avoid distractions and relax. Leave the television off and take a leisurely half-hour walk to remove the stress of the day. Just stay busy, and your future will be much brighter with a much healthier outlook.

BREAKFAST

1. Sweet Potatoes with Coconut Flakes

Preparation time: 15 minutes
Cooking time: 1 hour
Servings: 2
INGREDIENTS:

- 16 oz. sweet potatoes   • 1 tbsp. maple syrup
- ¼ c.
- Fat-free coconut Greek yogurt
- 1/8 c. unsweetened toasted coconut flakes
- 1 chopped apple   **DIRECTIONS:**
1. Preheat oven to 400 0F.
2. Place your potatoes on a baking sheet. Bake them for 45 - 60 minutes or until soft.
3. Use a sharp knife to mark "X" on the potatoes and fluff pulp with a fork.
4. Top with coconut flakes, chopped apple, Greek yogurt, and maple syrup.
5. Serve immediately.

NUTRITION: Calories: 321 Fat: 3 g Carbs: 70 g Protein: 7 g

2. Flaxseed & Banana Smoothie

Preparation time: 5 minutes
Cooking time: 0
Servings: 1
INGREDIENTS:

- 1 frozen banana ½ c. almond milk
- Vanilla extract. 1 tbsp. almond butter
- 2 tbsps. Flax seed 1 tsp. maple syrup   **DIRECTIONS:**
1. Sum up all your ingredients to a food processor or blender and run until smooth. Pour the mixture into a glass and enjoy.

NUTRITION: Calories: 376, Fat: 19.4 g Carbs: 48.3 g Protein: 9.2 g

3. Fruity Tofu Smoothie

Preparation time: 5 minutes
Cooking time: 0
Servings: 2
INGREDIENTS:

- 1 c. ice cold water
- 1 c. packed spinach
- ¼ c. frozen mango chunks

- ½ c. frozen pineapple chunks
- 1 tbsp. chia seeds
- 1 container silken tofu
- 1 frozen medium banana   **DIRECTIONS:**

1. In a mixer, add all ingredients and purée until smooth and creamy.
2. Evenly divide into two glasses, serve and enjoy.

NUTRITION: Calories: 175 Fat: 3.7 g Carbs: 33.3 g Protein: 6.0 g

4. French toast with Applesauce

Preparation time: 5 minutes
Cooking time: 5
Servings: 6
INGREDIENTS:
- ¼ c. unsweetened applesauce
- ½ c. skim milk
- 2 packets Stevia
- 2 eggs
- 6 slices whole wheat bread
- 1 tsp. ground cinnamon   **DIRECTIONS:**

1. Mix well applesauce, sugar, cinnamon, milk and eggs in a mixing bowl.
2. One slice, soak the bread into applesauce mixture until wet.
3. On medium fire, heat a large nonstick skillet.
4. Add soaked bread on one side and another on the other side. Cook in a single layer in batches for 2-3 minutes per side on medium low fire or until lightly browned.
5. Serve and enjoy.

NUTRITION: Calories: 122.6, Fat: 2.6 g Carbs: 18.3 g Protein: 6.5 g

5. Banana-Peanut Butter 'n Greens Smoothie

Preparation time: 5 minutes
Cooking time: 0
Servings: 1
INGREDIENTS:
- 1 c. chopped and packed Romaine lettuce
- 1 frozen medium banana
- 1 tbsp. all-natural peanut butter
- 1 c. cold almond milk   **DIRECTIONS:**

1. In a heavy-duty blender, add all ingredients.
2. Puree until smooth and creamy.
3. Serve and enjoy.

NUTRITION: Calories: 349.3, Fat: 9.7 g Carbs: 57.4 g Protein: 8.1 g

6. Baking Powder Biscuits

Preparation time: 5 minutes
Cooking time: 5 minutes
Servings: 1
INGREDIENTS:

- 1 egg white
- 1 c. white whole-wheat flour
- 4 tbsps. Non-hydrogenated vegetable shortening
- 1 tbsp. sugar
- 2/3 c. low- • Fat milk
- 1 c. unbleached all-purpose flour
- 4 tsps.
- Sodium-free baking powder   **DIRECTIONS:**
1. Preheat the oven to 450°F and leave the baking sheet aside.
2. Place the flour, sugar, and baking powder into a mixing bowl and whisk well to combine.
3. Break the shortening into the paste with your fingers, then work until it appears like hard crumbs. Attach the white egg and milk and stir to mix.
4. Let the dough out onto a lightly floured surface and knead for 1 minute. Roll the dough to 3/4 inch thickness and cut it into 12 rounds.
5. Place rounds on the baking sheet. Place baking sheet on middle rack in oven and bake 10 minutes.
6. Remove the baking sheet and put the cookies on the wire rack to cool.
   NUTRITION: Calories: 118, Fat: 4 g Carbs: 16 g Protein: 3 g

7. Oatmeal Banana Pancakes with Walnuts

Preparation time: 15 minutes
Cooking time: 5 minutes
Servings: 8 pancakes
INGREDIENTS:

- 1 finely diced firm banana
- 1 c. whole wheat pancake mix
- 1/8 c. chopped walnuts
- ¼ c. old-fashioned oats   **DIRECTIONS:**
1. Choose the pancake mix according to the directions on the package.
2. Add walnuts, oats, and chopped banana.
3. Coat a griddle with cooking spray. Add about ¼ cup of the pancake batter onto the griddle when hot.
4. Turn pancake over when bubbles form on top. Cook until golden brown.
5. Serve immediately.

NUTRITION: Calories: 155 Fat: 4 g Carbs: 28 g Protein: 7 g

8. Creamy Oats, Greens & Blueberry Smoothie

Preparation time: 4 minutes
Cooking time: 0
Servings: 1
INGREDIENTS:

- 1 c. cold
- Fat-free milk
- 1 c. salad greens
- ½ c. fresh frozen blueberries
- ½ c. frozen cooked oatmeal
- 1 tbsp. sunflower seeds   **DIRECTIONS:**

1. Blend all ingredients until smooth and creamy.
2. Serve and enjoy.

NUTRITION: Calories: 280, Fat: 6.8 g Carbs: 44.0 g Protein: 14.0 g

9. Banana & Cinnamon Oatmeal

Preparation time: 5 minutes
Cooking time: 0
Servings: 6
INGREDIENTS:

- 2 c. quick-cooking oats
- 4 c. Fat-free milk
- 1 tsp. ground cinnamon
- 2 chopped large ripe banana
- 4 tsps. Brown sugar
- Extra ground cinnamon   **DIRECTIONS:**

1. Place milk in a skillet and bring to boil. Add oats and cook over medium heat until thickened, for two to four minutes. Stir intermittently.
2. Add cinnamon, brown sugar and banana and stir to combine.
3. If you want, serve with the extra cinnamon and milk.   Enjoy!

NUTRITION: Calories: 215, Fat: 2 g Carbs: 42 g Protein: 10 g

LUNCH

10. Tomato and Halloumi Platter

Preparation time: 5 minutes
Cooking time: 4 minutes
Servings: 4
INGREDIENTS:

- 1 pound tomatoes, sliced
- ½ pound halloumi, cut into 4 slices

- 2 tablespoons parsley, chopped
- 1 tablespoon basil, chopped
- 2 tablespoons olive oil
- A pinch of salt and black pepper
- Juice of 1 lemon **DIRECTIONS:**

1. Brush the halloumi slices with half of the oil, put them on your preheated grill and cook over medium-high heat and cook for 2 minutes on each side.
2. Arrange the tomato slices on a platter, season with salt and pepper, drizzle the lemon juice and the rest of the oil all over, top with the halloumi slices, sprinkle the herbs on top and serve for lunch.

NUTRITION: Calories 181 Fat 7.3, fiber 1.4 Carbs 4.6 Protein 1.1

11. Chickpeas and Millet Stew

Preparation time: 10 minutes
Cooking time: 1 hour and 5 minutes
Servings: 4
INGREDIENTS:
- 1 cup millet
- 2 tablespoons olive oil
- A pinch of salt and black pepper
- 1 eggplant, cubed
- 1 yellow onion, chopped
- 14 ounces canned tomatoes, chopped
- 14 ounces canned chickpeas, drained and rinsed
- 3 garlic cloves, minced
- 2 tablespoons harissa paste
- 1 bunch cilantro, chopped
- 2 cups water **DIRECTIONS:**

1. Put the water in a pan, bring to a simmer over medium heat, add the millet, simmer for 25 minutes, take off the heat, fluff with a fork and leave aside for now.
2. Heat a pan with half of the oil over medium heat, add the eggplant, salt and pepper, stir, cook for 10 minutes and transfer to a bowl.
3. Add the rest of the oil to the pan, heat up over medium heat again, add the onion and sauté for 10 minutes.
4. Add the garlic, more salt and pepper, the harrisa, chickpeas, tomatoes and return the eggplant, stir and cook over low heat for 15 minutes more.
5. Add the millet, toss, divide the mix into bowls, sprinkle the cilantro on top and serve.

NUTRITION: Calories 671 Fat 15.6 Carbs 87.5 Protein 27.1

12. Chicken Salad

Preparation time: 30 minutes
Cooking time: 45 minutes
Servings: 4
INGREDIENTS:

- 1 and ½ pounds chicken breast, skinless, boneless
- 1 tablespoon dill, chopped
- Zest of 2 lemons, grated
- Juice of 2 lemons
- 3 tablespoons olive oil
- 1 tablespoon oregano, chopped
- 3 tablespoons parsley, chopped • A pinch of salt and black pepper
- For the barley:
- 2 and ½ cups chicken stock
- 1 cup barley
- 1 teaspoon oregano, dried
- Zest of 1 lemon, grated
- Juice of 1 lemon
- ¼ cup olive oil
- 2 red leaf lettuce heads, chopped
- 1 red onion, sliced
- 1 pint cherry tomatoes, sliced
- 2 avocados, peeled, pitted and sliced **DIRECTIONS:**
   1. Put the chicken breasts in a bowl, add the dill, zest of 2 lemons, juice of 2 lemons, 3 tablespoons oil, 1 tablespoon oregano, parsley, salt and pepper, toss, cover the bowl and leave aside for 30 minutes.
   2. Heat your grill over medium-high heat, add the chicken, cook for 6 minutes on each side, cool down, slice and put in a bowl.
   3. Put the stock in a pot, add the barley, salt and pepper, bring to a simmer over medium heat, cook for 45 minutes, drain and put in the same bowl with the chicken.
   4. Add the dried oregano, zest of 1 lemon, juice of 1 lemon, ¼ cup oil, the lettuce, onion, tomatoes and the avocados, toss and serve. **NUTRITION:** Calories 342 Fat 17.4 Carbs 27.7 Protein 26.4

13. Chicken Skillet

Preparation time: 10 minutes
Cooking time: 35 minutes
Servings: 6
INGREDIENTS:

- 6 chicken thighs, bone-in and skin-on
- Juice of 2 lemons
- 1 teaspoon oregano, dried

- 1 red onion, chopped
- Salt and black pepper to the taste
- 1 teaspoon garlic powder
- 2 garlic cloves, minced
- 2 tablespoons olive oil
- 2 and ½ cups chicken stock
- 1 cup white rice
- 1 tablespoon oregano, chopped
- 1 cup green olives, pitted and sliced
- 1/3 cup parsley, chopped
- ½ cup feta cheese, crumbled **DIRECTIONS:**

1. Heat a pan with the oil over medium heat, add the chicken thighs skin side down, cook for 4 minutes on each side and transfer to a plate.
2. Add the garlic and the onion to the pan, stir and sauté for 5 minutes.
3. Add the rice, salt, pepper, the stock, oregano, and lemon juice, stir, cook for 1-2 minutes more and take off the heat.
4. Add the chicken to the pan, introduce the pan in the oven and bake at 375 degrees F for 25 minutes.
5. Add the cheese, olives and the parsley, divide the whole mix between plates and serve for lunch.

NUTRITION: Calories 435 Fat 18.5 Carbs 27.8 Protein 25.6

14. Tuna and Couscous

Preparation time: 10 minutes
Cooking time: 0 minutes
Servings: 4
INGREDIENTS:

- 1 cup chicken stock
- 1 and ¼ cups couscous
- A pinch of salt and black pepper
- 10 ounces canned tuna, drained and flaked
- 1 pint cherry tomatoes, halved
- ½ cup pepperoncini, sliced
- 1/3 cup parsley, chopped
- 1 tablespoon olive oil
- ¼ cup capers, drained
- Juice of ½ lemon **DIRECTIONS:**

1. Put the stock in a pan, bring to a boil over medium-high heat, add the couscous, stir, take off the heat, cover, leave aside for 10 minutes, fluff with a fork and transfer to a bowl.
2. Add the tuna and the rest of the ingredients, toss and serve for lunch right away.

NUTRITION: Calories 253 Fat 11.5 Carbs 16.5 Protein 23.2

15. Chicken Stuffed Peppers

Preparation time: 10 minutes
Cooking time: 0 minutes
Servings: 6
INGREDIENTS:

- 1 cup Greek yogurt
- 2 tablespoons mustard
- Salt and black pepper to the taste
- 1 pound rotisserie chicken meat, cubed
- 4 celery stalks, chopped
- 2 tablespoons balsamic vinegar
- 1 bunch scallions, sliced
- ¼ cup parsley, chopped
- 1 cucumber, sliced
- 3 red bell peppers, halved and deseeded
- 1 pint cherry tomatoes, quartered **DIRECTIONS:**

1. Add the chicken in a bowl with the celery and the rest of the ingredients except the bell peppers and toss well.
2. Stuff the peppers halves with the chicken mix and serve for lunch.

NUTRITION: Calories 266 Fat 12.2 Carbs 15.7 Protein 3.7

16. Turkey Fritters and Sauce

Preparation time: 10 minutes
Cooking time: 30 minutes
Servings: 4
INGREDIENTS:

- 2 garlic cloves, minced
- 1 egg
- 1 red onion, chopped
- 1 tablespoon olive oil
- ¼ teaspoon red pepper flakes
- 1 pound turkey meat, ground
- ½ teaspoon oregano, dried • Cooking spray
- For the sauce:
- 1 cup Greek yogurt
- 1 cucumber, chopped
- 1 tablespoon olive oil
- ¼ teaspoon garlic powder
- 2 tablespoons lemon juice
- ¼ cup parsley, chopped **DIRECTIONS:**

1. Heat a pan with 1 tablespoon oil over medium heat, add the onion and the garlic, sauté for 5 minutes, cool down and transfer to a bowl.
2. Add the meat, turkey, oregano and pepper flakes, stir and shape medium patties out of this mix.
3. Heat another pan greased with cooking spray over medium-high heat, add the turkey patties and brown for 5 minutes on each side.
4. Introduce the pan in the oven and bake the cakes at 375 degrees F for 15 minutes more.
5. Meanwhile, in a bowl, mix the yogurt with the cucumber, oil, garlic powder, lemon juice and parsley and whisk well.
6. Divide the fritters between plates, spread the sauce all over and serve for lunch.

NUTRITION: Calories 364 Fat 16.8 Carbs 26.8 Protein 23.4

17. Stuffed Eggplants

Preparation time: 10 minutes
Cooking time: 35 minutes
Servings: 4
INGREDIENTS:

- 2 eggplants, halved lengthwise and 2/3 of the flesh scooped out
- 3 tablespoons olive oil
- 1 red onion, chopped
- 2 garlic cloves, minced
- 1 pint white mushrooms, sliced
- 2 cups kale, torn
- 2 cups quinoa, cooked
- 1 tablespoon thyme, chopped
- Zest and juice of 1 lemon
- Salt and black pepper to the taste
- ½ cup Greek yogurt
- 3 tablespoons parsley, chopped   **DIRECTIONS:**

1. Rub the inside of each eggplant half with half of the oil and put on a baking sheet lined with parchment paper.
2. Heat a pan with the rest of the oil over medium heat, add the onion and the garlic and sauté for 5 minutes.
3. Add the mushrooms and cook for 5 minutes more.
4. Add the kale, salt, pepper, thyme, lemon zest and juice, stir, cook for 5 minutes more and take off the heat.
5. Stuff the eggplant halves with the mushroom mix, introduce them in the oven and bake 400 degrees F for 20 minutes.
6. Divide the eggplants between plates, sprinkle the parsley and the yogurt on top and serve for lunch.

NUTRITION: Calories 512 Fat 16.4 Carbs 78 Protein 17.2

18. Salmon Bowls

Preparation time: 10 minutes
Cooking time: 40 minutes
Servings: 4
INGREDIENTS:

- 2 cups farro
- Juice of 2 lemons
- 1/3 cup olive oil+ 2 tablespoons
- Salt and black pepper
- 1 cucumber, chopped
- ¼ cup balsamic vinegar
- 1 garlic cloves, minced
- ¼ cup parsley, chopped
- ¼ cup mint, chopped
- 2 tablespoons mustard
- 4 salmon fillets, boneless **DIRECTIONS:**

1. Put the water in a big pot, bring to a boil over medium-high heat, add salt and flour, stir, simmer for 30 minutes, rinse, move to a bowl, add the lemon juice, mustard, garlic, salt, pepper and 1/3 cup of oil, toss and set aside for now.
2. In another bowl, mash the cucumber with a fork, add the vinegar, salt, pepper, the parsley, dill and mint and whisk well.
3. Heat up a pan with the rest of the oil over medium heat, add the salmon fillets skin side down, cook for 5 minutes on each side, cool them down and break into pieces.
4. Add over the farro, add the cucumber dressing, toss and serve for lunch.
NUTRITION: Calories 281 Fat 12.7 Carbs 5.8 Protein 36.5

APPETIZERS

19. Greek Yogurt (Used as Dip)

Preparation time: 5 minutes
Cooking time: 0 minutes
Servings: 1
INGREDIENTS:

- 6 oz. Greek yogurt (plain and fat-free kind)
- ¼ cup crumbled tomato-basil feta cheese
- 2 tbsp. Reduced-fat mayonnaise
- 2tbsp chopped fresh parsley
- Assorted fresh vegetables **DIRECTIONS:**

1. Mix yogurt, cheese, mayonnaise, and parsley in a small bowl. Divide the dip among bowls and serve with your favorite vegetables. **NUTRITION:** Calories: 50 Carbs: 4g Fat: 4g Protein: 2g

20. Lemon Garlic Sesame Hummus Dip

Preparation time: 5 minutes
Cooking time: 0 minutes
Servings: 1
INGREDIENTS:

- Tahini, lemon juice (fresh squeezed) • 2 tbsp. Extra virgin olive oil
- 2 tbsp. toasted white sesame seeds
- 3 peeled and crushed garlic cloves
- 15 ounces drained garbanzo beans (reserve liquid)
- 1 ½ tbsp. minced lemon peel
- 1 tbsp. minced orange peel
- Sea salt
- White pepper **DIRECTIONS:**

1. Combine sesame seeds, extra virgin olive oil, garlic, garbanzo beans (reserve 1 tablespoon for garnish), lemon juice, and tahini in a food processor.
2. Keep adding the garbanzo bean liquid only if it is necessary until desired consistency.
3. Season hummus with sea salt and pepper and garnish with the reserved beans, and sprinkle with lemon and orange peel. Refrigerate until chilled. **NUTRITION:** Calories: 60 Carbs: 6g Fat: 3g Protein: 2g

21. Creamy Greek Yogurt and Cucumber

Preparation time: 5 minutes
Cooking time: 0 minutes
Servings: 1
INGREDIENTS:

- 2 English cucumbers, thinly sliced
- Small bunch dill
- 1 ½ cups low-fat Greek yogurt
- 2 tbsp. Fresh lemon juice
- 1 ½ tsp. mustard seeds
- Coarse salt and ground pepper **DIRECTIONS:**

1. Combine all your fixings in a bowl until combined well and dig in!
NUTRITION: Calories: 21 Carbs: 2g Fat: 0g Protein: 23g

22. Nachos

Preparation time: 5 minutes

Cooking time: 10 minutes
Servings: 4
INGREDIENTS:

- 4-ounce restaurant-style corn tortilla chips
- 1 medium green onion, thinly sliced (about 1 tbsp.)
- 1 (4 ounces) package finely crumbled feta cheese
- 1 finely chopped and drained plum tomato
- 2 tbsp. Sun-dried tomatoes in oil, finely chopped
- 2 tbsp. Kalamata olives   **DIRECTIONS:**

1. Mix an onion, plum tomato, oil, sun-dried tomatoes, and olives in a small bowl.
2. Arrange the tortillas chips on a microwavable plate in a single layer topped evenly with cheese—microwave on high for one minute.
3. Rotate the plate half turn and continue microwaving until the cheese is bubbly. Spread the tomato mixture over the chips and cheese and enjoy.

NUTRITION: Calories: 140 Carbs: 19g Fat: 7g Protein: 2g

23. Stuffed Celery

Preparation time: 15 minutes
Cooking time: 20 minutes
Servings: 3
INGREDIENTS:

- Olive oil
- 1 clove garlic, minced
- 2 tbsp. Pine nuts
- 2 tbsp. dry-roasted sunflower seeds
- ¼ cup Italian cheese blend, shredded
- 8 stalks celery leaves
- 1 (8-ounce) fat-free cream cheese
- Cooking spray   **DIRECTIONS:**

1. Sauté garlic and pine nuts over a medium setting for the heat until the nuts are golden brown. Cut off the broad base and tops from celery.
2. Remove two thin strips from the round side of the celery to create a flat surface.
3. Mix Italian cheese and cream cheese in a bowl and spread into cut celery stalks.
4. Sprinkle half of the celery pieces with sunflower seeds and a half with the pine nut mixture. Cover mixture and let stand for at least 4 hours before eating.

NUTRITION: Calories: 64 Carbs: 2g Fat: 6g Protein: 1g

24. Butternut Squash Fries

Preparation time: 5 minutes
Cooking time: 10 minutes
Servings: 2
INGREDIENTS:

- 1 Butternut squash
- 1 tbsp. Extra virgin olive oil
- ½ tbsp. Grape seed oil
- 1/8 tsp. Sea salt   **DIRECTIONS:**

1. Remove seeds from the squash and cut them into thin slices. Coat with extra virgin olive oil and grape seed oil. Add a sprinkle of salt and toss to coat well.
2. Arrange the squash slices onto three baking sheets and bake for 10 minutes until crispy.

NUTRITION: Calories: 40 Carbs: 10g Fat: 0g Protein: 1g

25. Dried Fig Tapenade

Preparation time: 5 minutes
Cooking time: 0 minutes
Servings: 1
INGREDIENTS:

- 1 cup Dried figs
- 1 cup Kalamata olives
- ½ cup Water
- 1 tbsp. Chopped fresh thyme
- 1 tbsp. extra virgin olive oil
- ½ tsp. Balsamic vinegar   **DIRECTIONS:**

1. Prepare figs in a food processor until well chopped, add water, and continue processing to form a paste.
2. Add olives and pulse until well blended. Add thyme, vinegar, and extra virgin olive oil and pulse until very smooth. Best served with crackers of your choice.
NUTRITION: Calories: 249 Carbs: 64g Fat: 1g Protein: 3g

26. Speedy Sweet Potato Chips

Preparation time: 15 minutes
Cooking time: 60 minutes
Servings: 4
INGREDIENTS:

- 1 large Sweet potato
- 1 tbsp. Extra virgin olive oil
- Salt

DIRECTIONS:

1. 300°F preheated oven. Slice your potato into nice, thin slices that resemble fries.
2. Toss the potato slices with salt and extra virgin olive oil in a bowl. Bake for about one hour, flipping every 15 minutes until crispy and browned.   **NUTRITION:** Calories: 150 Carbs: 16g Fat: 9g Protein: 1g

27. Nachos with Hummus (Mediterranean Inspired)

Preparation time: 15 minutes
Cooking time: 20 minutes
Servings: 4
INGREDIENTS:

- 4 cups salted pita chips
- 1 (8 oz.) red pepper (roasted)
- Hummus
- 1 tsp. Finely shredded lemon peel
- ¼ cup Chopped pitted Kalamata olives
- ¼ cup crumbled feta cheese
- 1 plum (Roma) tomato, seeded, chopped
- ½ cup chopped cucumber
- 1 tsp. Chopped fresh oregano leaves   **DIRECTIONS:**

1. 400°F preheated oven. Arrange the pita chips on a heatproof platter and drizzle with hummus.
2. Top with olives, tomato, cucumber, and cheese and bake until warmed .Sprinkle lemon zest and oregano and enjoy while it's hot.

NUTRITION: Calories: 130 Carbs: 18g Fat: 5g Protein: 4g

28. Pineapple Mediterranean Dip

Preparation time: 5 minutes
Cooking time: 0 minutes
Servings: 1
INGREDIENTS:

- 16 strawberries
- 8 bunches grapes
- 2 nectarines, thinly sliced
- 1 can pineapple (drained)
- Flaked and toasted coconut (¼ cup)
- Choc chip cookies   **DIRECTIONS:**

1. Mix a pineapple, coconut, and yogurt in a bowl and top with fruit and cookies. Cover and refrigerate for one hour before eating.

NUTRITION: Calories: 100 Carbs: 0g Fat: 2g Protein: 2g

29. Mediterranean Inspired Tapenade

Preparation time: 5 minutes
Cooking time: 0 minutes
Servings: 1
INGREDIENTS:

- 1 cup Pitted Kalamata olives

- 5 cloves garlic
- One lemon, juiced
- 2 tbsp. Extra virgin olive oil
- 1 tbsp. capers
- ½ tsp. Allspice
- ¼ cup Chopped parsley   **DIRECTIONS:**

1. Process all fixings using a food processor until blended well. Serve and enjoy!

NUTRITION: Calories: 80 Carbs: 2g Fat: 7g Protein: 0g

SALADS

30. Lentil Salmon Salad

Preparation time: 25 minutes
Cooking time: 0
Servings 4
INGREDIENTS

- Vegetable stock - 2 cups
- Green lentils - 1, rinsed
- Red onion - 1, chopped
- Parsley - 1 2 cup, chopped
- Smoked salmon - 4 oz., shredded
- Cilantro - 2 tbsp., chopped
- Red pepper - 1, chopped
- Lemon - 1, juiced
- Salt and pepper - to taste

DIRECTIONS

1. Cook vegetable stock and lentils in a saucepan for 15 to 20 minutes, on low heat. Ensure all liquid has been absorbed and then remove from heat.
2. Pour into a salad bowl and top with red pepper, parsley, cilantro, salt and pepper (to suit your taste) and mix.
3. Mix in lemon juice and shredded salmon.
4. Serve fresh.

NUTRITION: Calories: 300 Fat: 17 Carb: 24 Protein: 20

31. Peppy Pepper Tomato Salad

Preparation time: 20 minutes
Cookingtime:0
Servings 4
INGREDIENTS

- Yellow bell pepper - 1, cored and diced

- Cucumbers - 4, diced
- Red onion - 1, chopped   • Balsamic vinegar – 1 tbsp.
- oil – 2 tbsp.
- Tomatoes - 4, diced
- Red bell peppers - 2, cored and diced
- Chili flakes - 1 pinch
- Salt and pepper - to taste   **DIRECTIONS:**

1. Mix the ingredients in a salad bowl, except salt and pepper.
2. Season with salt and pepper to suit your taste and mix well.
3. Eat while fresh.

NUTRITION: Calories: 163 Fat: 3 Fiber: 17 Protein: 4.5

32. Bulgur Salad

Preparation time: 30 minutes
Cooking time: 0
Servings 4
INGREDIENTS
- Vegetable stock - 2 cups
- Bulgur - 2 3 cup
- Garlic clove - 1, minced
- Cherry tomatoes - 1 cup, halved
- Almonds - 2 tbsp., sliced
- Dates - 1 4 cup • Lemon juice - 1 tbsp.
- Baby spinach - 8 oz.
- Cucumber - 1, diced   • Balsamic vinegar - 1 tbsp.
- Salt and pepper - to taste

DIRECTIONS
1. Pour the vegetable stock into a saucepan and heat until hot, then stir in bulgur and cook until bulgur has absorbed all stock.
2. Put in a salad bowl and add remaining ingredients: stir well.
3. Season with salt and pepper that will suit your taste.
4. Serve and eat immediately.

NUTRITION: Calories: 151 Carbs: 34 grams Protein: 6 grams Fat: 0 grams Fiber: 8 grams

33. Tasty Tuna Salad

Preparation Time: 15 minutes
Cooking time: 0
Servings 4
INGREDIENTS
- Green olives - 1 4 cups, sliced   • Tuna in water - 1 can drain

- Pine nuts - 2 tbsp.
- Artichoke hearts – 1 jar, drained and chopped • oil - 2 tbsp.
- Lemon – 1, juiced
- Arugula - 2 leaves • Dijon mustard - 1 tbsp.
- Salt and pepper - to taste

DIRECTIONS

1. In a cup, combine the mustard, oil and lemon juice to create a dressing.
2. Combine the artichoke hearts, tuna, green olives, arugula, and pine nuts in a salad bowl.
3. In a separate salad bowl, mix tuna, arugula, pine nuts, artichoke hearts, and tuna.
4. Pour dressing mix onto the salad and serve fresh.

NUTRITION: Calories: 251.3 Total Fat: 13.4 g Protein: 25.4 g Saturated Fat: 25 g

34. Sweet and Sour Spinach Salad

Preparation Time: 15 minutes
Cooking time: 0
Servings 4

INGREDIENTS

- Red onions - 2, sliced
- Baby spinach leaves - 4
- Sesame oil - 1 2 tsp.
- Apple cider vinegar - 2 tbsp.
- Honey - 1 tsp.
- Sesame seeds - 2 tbsp.
- Salt and pepper - to taste

DIRECTIONS

1. Mix honey, sesame oil, vinegar, and sesame seeds in a small bowl for dressing
2. Season with salt and pepper that will suit your taste.
3. Add red onions and spinach together in a salad bowl.
4. Pour dressing over the salad and serve while cool and fresh.

NUTRITION: Calories: 234 Crab: 23 Protein: 8.7 Fat: 13

35. Easy Eggplant Salad

Preparation time: 30 minutes
Cooking time: 0
Servings 4

INGREDIENTS

- Salt and pepper - to taste
- Eggplant - 2, sliced

- Smoked paprika - 1 tsp.
- Extra virgin olive oil - 2 tbsp.
- Garlic cloves - 2, minced
- Mixed greens - 2 cups   • Sherry vinegar - 2 tbsp.

DIRECTIONS

1. Mix garlic, paprika, and oil in a small bowl.
2. Place eggplant on a plate and sprinkle with salt and pepper to suit your taste. Next, brush the oil mixture onto the eggplant.
3. Cook eggplant on a medium heated grill pan until brown on both sides. Once cooked, put eggplant into a salad bowl.
4. Top with greens and vinegar, serve and eat.

NUTRITION: Calories: 150.5 Total Fat: 10.9 g Dietary Fiber: 4.9 g Saturated Fat: 1.5 g

36. Sweetest Sweet Potato Salad

Preparation Time: 15 minutes
Cooking time: 15 minutes
Servings 4
INGREDIENTS

- Honey - 2 tbsp.
- Sumac spice - 1 tsp.
- Sweet potato - 2, finely sliced
- Extra virgin olive oil - 3 tbsp.
- Dried mint - 1 tsp.
- Balsamic vinegar – 1 tbsp.
- Salt and pepper - to taste
- Pomegranate - 1, seeded
- Mixed greens - 3 cups

DIRECTIONS

1. Place sweet potato slices on a plate and add sumac, mint, salt, and pepper on both sides. Next, drizzle oil and honey over both sides.
2. Add oil to a grill pan and heat. Grill sweet potatoes on medium heat until brown on both sides.
3. Put sweet potatoes in a salad bowl and top with pomegranate and mixed greens.
4. Stir and eat right away.

NUTRITION: 244 calories Protein 4.9g Carbohydrates 14.3g Fat 19g Cholesterol 100.8mg Sodium 480.7mg

SOUPS & STEWS RECIPES

37. Italian Broccoli & Potato Soup

Preparation time: 5 minutes
Cooking Time: 45 Minutes
Servings: 4
INGREDIENTS:

- 1 lb. broccoli, cut into florets
- 2 potatoes, peeled, chopped
- 4 cups vegetable broth
- ½ tsp. dried rosemary
- ½ tsp. salt
- ½ cup sour cream **DIRECTIONS:**

1. Place broccoli and potatoes in the pot. Pour the broth and seal the lid. Cook on Soup/Broth for 20 minutes on High. Do a quick release and remove to a blender. Pulse to combine. Stir in sour cream and add salt.

NUTRITION: Calories: 239kcal Carbohydrates: 25.5g Protein: 16g, Fat: 9.5g Saturated Fat: 5g Cholesterol: 30mg Sodium: 603mg Fiber: 3.5g

38. Broccoli Soup with Gorgonzola

Preparation time: 5 minutes
Cooking Time: 35 Minutes
Servings: 4
INGREDIENTS:

- 8 oz. Gorgonzola cheese, crumbled
- 1 cup broccoli, finely chopped
- 4 cups water
- 1 tbsp. olive oil
- ½ cup full-fat milk
- 1 tbsp. parsley, finely chopped
- ½ tsp. salt
- ¼ tsp. black pepper, ground **DIRECTIONS:**

1. Add all ingredients to the pot, seal the lid and cook on Soup/Broth mode for 30 minutes on High Pressure. Do a quick release. Remove the cover and sprinkle with fresh parsley. Serve warm.

NUTRITION: 210Cal 9gCarbs 16gFat 8gProtein

39. Comfort Food Soup

Preparation time: 10 minutes
Cooking Time: 30 Minutes

Servings: 8
INGREDIENTS:

- 1 C. yellow split peas
- 1 C. red lentils
- 1 large onion, chopped roughly
- 2 carrots, peeled and chopped roughly
- 5 garlic cloves, chopped
- 1½ tsp. ground cumin
- Salt and freshly ground black pepper
- 8 C. chicken broth
- 2 tbsp. fresh lemon juice **DIRECTIONS:**

1. In the pot of Instant Pot, place all the ingredients except for lemon juice.
2. Secure the lid and put the pressure valve on the "Seal"
3. Choose "Manual" and cook under "High Pressure" for about 30 minutes.
4. Select "Cancel" and do a "Natural" release.
5. Remove the lid and stir in lemon juice.
6. Serve hot.

NUTRITION: Calories 226 Carbohydrates: 34.3g Protein: 17.7g Fat: 2.1g Sugar: 4.8g Sodium: 801mg Fiber: 14.5g

40. Comfy Meal Stew

Preparation time: 15 minutes
Cooking Time: 1 Hour 6
Minutes **Servings:** 6
INGREDIENTS:

- ¼ C. flour
- Salt and freshly ground black pepper
- 2 lb. lamb shoulder, cut into 1-inch cubes
- 2 tbsp. olive oil
- ½ C. celery, chopped
- ½ C. carrots, peeled and chopped
- ½ C. fennel, chopped
- ½ C. leeks, sliced
- 1 tsp. dried rosemary, crushed
- 2 tbsp. brandy
- 1 (28-oz.) can diced tomatoes
- 1 (15-oz.) can chickpeas, drained and rinsed
- 2 C. beef broth
- 1 bay leaf
- 2 tbsp. fresh parsley, chopped **DIRECTIONS:**

1. Mix the flour in a large bowl, salt, and black pepper.
2. Add the lamb cubes and toss to coat well.

3. Place the oil in Instant Pot and select "Sauté." Then add the lamb cubes in 2 batches and cook for about 4-5 minutes.
4. With a slotted spoon, transfer the lamb cubes into a bowl.
5. In the pot, add the celery, carrots, fennel and cook for about 5 minutes.
6. Stir in the rosemary and brandy and cook for about 1 minute, scraping up any browned bits from the bottom.
7. Select "Cancel" and stir in the cooked lamb cubes, tomatoes, chickpeas, broth, and bay leaf.
8. Secure the lid and put the pressure valve in the location of the "Seal." 9. "Pick "Manual" and cook for about 45 minutes under "High Pressure".Select "Cancel" and do a "Natural" release.
10.   Remove the lid and serve hot with the garnishing of parsley.

NUTRITION: Calories: 478 Carbohydrates: 28.5g Protein: 49.7g Fat: 17.4g Sugar: 4.6g Sodium: 634mg Fiber: 5.7g

41. Exciting Chickpeas Soup

Preparation time: 2 minutes
Cooking Time: 8 Minutes
Servings: 6
INGREDIENTS:

- 2 tbsp. olive oil
- 1 C. onion, chopped
- 4-5 garlic cloves, crushed
- 1 C. carrot, peeled and chopped
- 1 C. celery stalk, chopped
- 2 (15½ oz.) cans chickpeas, drained and rinsed
- 1 (14½ oz.) can fire-roasted tomatoes
- 2 tbsp. tomato paste
- 1 tbsp. sun-dried tomatoes
- ½ tsp. ground cinnamon
- 2 tsp. ground cumin
- 2 tsp. paprika
- 2 tsp. ground coriander
- Salt and freshly ground black pepper
- 4 C. vegetable broth
- 2 C. fresh baby spinach, chopped
- 1 tbsp. fresh lemon juice **DIRECTIONS:**

1. Place the ingredients except the spinach and lemon juice in the Instant Pot pot and mix to combine
2. "Pick "Manual" and cook for around 8 minutes under "High Pressure".
3. Select "Cancel" and do a "Natural" release for about 10 minutes, then do a "Quick" release.

4. Remove the lid, and with a potato masher, mash some beans.
5. Stir in
6. spinach juice and lemon juice and set aside for about 5 minutes before eating.

NUTRITION: Calories: 35 Carbohydrates: 50.5g Protein: 18.2g; Fat: 9.9g; Sugar: 12.1g; Sodium: 938mg; Fiber: 14g

42. Classic Napoli Sauce

Preparation time: 10 minutes
Cooking Time: 45 Minutes
Servings: 4
INGREDIENTS:

- 1 lb. mushrooms
- 2 cups canned tomatoes, diced
- 1 carrot, chopped
- 1 onion, chopped
- 1 celery stick, chopped
- 1 tbsp. olive oil
- 1 tsp. salt
- ½ tsp. paprika
- 1 tsp. fish sauce
- 1 cup water **DIRECTIONS:**

1. Steam the sautéed olive oil. For 5 minutes, stir-fry the carrot, onion, celery, and paprika. Add the ingredients, except the tomatoes, and cook for another 5-6 minutes, until the meat is lightly browned. Please seal the lid
2. Cook on High Pressure for 20 minutes. When done, release the steam naturally, for about 10 minutes. Hit Sauté, and cook for 7-8 minutes, to thicken the sauce.

NUTRITION: 61Cal 8gCarbs 2gFat 1gProtein

43. Winter Dinner Stew

Preparation time: 2 minutes
Cooking Time: 14 Minutes
Servings: 6
INGREDIENTS:

- 3 tbsp. extra-virgin olive oil
- 1 small onion, sliced thinly
- 1 small green bell peppe
- 1½ C. tomatoes, chopped
- 2 garlic cloves, minced
- ¼ C. fresh cilantro, chopped and divided
- 2 bay leaves
- 2 tsp. paprika
- Salt and freshly ground black pepper

- 1 C. fish broth
- 1 lb. shrimp, peeled and deveined
- 12 littleneck clams
- 1½ lb. cod fillets, cut into 2-inch chunks **DIRECTIONS:**

1. Place the oil in Instant Pot and select "Sauté." Then add the onion, bell pepper, tomatoes, garlic, 2 tbsp. Of cilantro, bay leaves, paprika, salt, and black pepper, and cook for about 3-4 minutes.
2. Select "Cancel" and stir in the broth.
3. Submerge the clams and shrimps into the vegetable mixture and top with the codpieces.
4. Secure the lid and put the pressure valve in the location of the "Seal."
5. Pick "Manual" and cook for about 10 minutes under "High Pressure."
6. Select "Cancel" and do a "Natural" release for about 10 minutes, then do a "Quick" release.
7. Remove the lid and serve hot with the garnishing of remaining cilantro.

NUTRITION: Calories: 450 Carbohydrates: 6.2g Protein: 79.3g **B** Fat: 11.9g Sugar: 2.8g Sodium: 487mg Fiber: 1.4g

44. Meatless-Monday Chickpeas Stew

Preparation time: 5 minutes
Cooking Time: 16 Minutes
Servings: 8
INGREDIENTS:

- ¼ C. olive oil
- 1 onion, chopped
- 7 garlic cloves, chopped finely
- 1 tsp. ground cinnamon
- 1½ tsp. ground cumin
- 2 tsp. sweet paprika
- 1/8 tsp. cayenne pepper
- 3 (14½ oz.) cans chickpeas, rinsed and drained
- 1 (14½ oz.) can diced tomatoes
- 1 C. carrots, peeled and chopped
- 4 C. low-sodium vegetable broth
- Salt and freshly ground black pepper
- 7 oz. fresh baby spinach **DIRECTIONS:**

1. Instant jar, put the oil and sauté. Add the onion and cook for about 3-4 minutes. Put the garlic and cook for about 1 minute.
2. Put some spices and cook for about 1 minute.
3. Select "Cancel" and stir in the chickpeas, diced tomatoes with juice, carrots, and broth.
4. Secure the lid and put the pressure valve in the location of the "Seal."

5. Pick "Manual" and cook for about 10 minutes under "High Pressure,".
6. Select "Cancel" and do a "Natural" release for about 15 minutes, then do a "Quick" release.
7. Remove the lid, and with a potato masher, mash the most of the stew.
8. Add the spinach and stir until wilted.
9. Serve immediately.

NUTRITION: Calorie: 279 Carbohydrates: 42.5g Protein: 10.4g Fat: 8.5g Sugar: 2.8g Sodium: 549mg Fiber: 9g

45. Fragrant Fish Stew

Preparation time: 3minutes
Cooking Time: 15 Minutes
Servings: 4
INGREDIENTS:
- 4 tbsp. extra-virgin olive oil, divided
- 1 medium red onion, sliced thinly
- 4 garlic cloves, chopped
- ½ C. dry white wine
- ½ lb. red potatoes, cubed
- 1 (15-oz.) can diced tomatoes with juices
- 1/8 tsp. red pepper flakes, crushed
- Salt and freshly ground black pepper
- 1 (8-oz.) bottled clam juice
- 2½ C. water
- 2 lb. sea bass, cut into 2-inch pieces
- 2 tbsp. fresh dill, chopped
- 2 tbsp. fresh lemon juice **DIRECTIONS:**

1. Location 2 tbsp. In Instant Pot, pick "Sauté." from the oil and then add the onion and cook for about 3 minutes. Add the garlic and simmer for about a minute.
2. Add the wine and cook for about 1 minute, scraping up any browned bits from the bottom.
3. Select "Cancel" and stir in the potatoes, tomatoes with juices, red pepper flakes, salt, black pepper, clam juice, and water.
4. Secure the lid and put the pressure valve in the location of the "Seal." 5. Choose "Manual" and cook under "High Pressure" for around 5 minutes..
6. Select "Cancel" and carefully do a "Quick" release.
7. Remove the lid and select "Sauté."
8. Stir in the fish pieces and cook for about 5 minutes.
9. Select "Cancel" and stir in the dill and lemon juice.
10. Serve hot.

NUTRITION: Calories: 533; Carbohydrates: 24.8g Protein: 56.8g Fat: 20.4g

Sugar: 6.9g Sodium: 458mg Fiber: 3.4g

SIDES

46. Artichoke Hearts

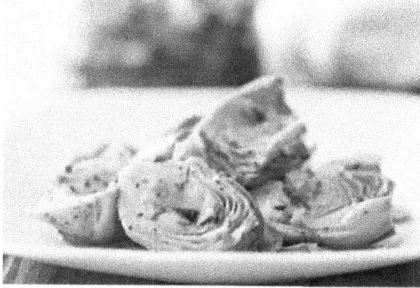

Preparation time: 10 minutes
Preparation Time: 30 Minute
Serves: 4
INGREDIENTS:

- ¾ Cup Cornmeal
- 1/3 cup Parmesan Cheese, Finely Grated
- 1 Teaspoon Garlic Powder
- 1 Teaspoon Sea Salt, Fine
- ½ Teaspoon Rosemary
- ½ Teaspoon Paprika
- ¼ Teaspoon Black Pepper
- 2 Eggs, Beaten Lightly
- ½ Cup Olive Oil, Divided
- 14 Ounces Artichoke Hearts, Canned & Drained **DIRECTIONS:**

1. Preheat your oven to 400, and then get out a wide but shallow bowl. In this bowl, combine your garlic, salt, rosemary, parmesan, paprika, and pepper. Make sure it's mixed well.
2. Mix your eggs and ¼ cup of olive oil. Drain your artichoke hearts and add them to the egg mixture, stirring to combine.
3. Get out a rimmed baking sheet and oil it with the remaining olive oil.
4. Remove your artichoke hearts from the egg mixture, and roll them in the cornmeal mixture until they. Place them on your baking sheet, and then bake for fifteen-twenty minutes. Serve hot.

NUTRITION: Calories: 415 Protein: 12 Grams Fat: 31 Grams Carbs: 29 Grams

47. Roasted Baby Potatoes

Preparation time: 5 minutes
Cooking Time: 45 Minutes
Serves: 4
INGREDIENTS:

- 2 lbs. Red Potatoes, Scrubbed & Cut into Wedges
- 1 Teaspoon Sweet Paprika
- 1 Teaspoon Garlic Powder
- 2 Teaspoon Rosemary, Fresh & chopped
- 2 Tablespoons Olive Oil
- ½ Teaspoon Sea Salt, Fine
- ½ Teaspoon Black Pepper

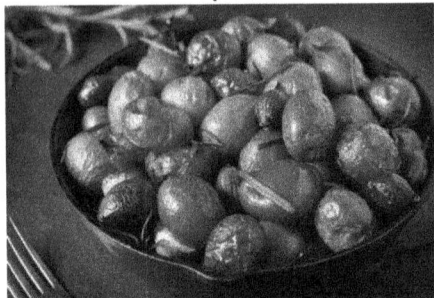

DIRECTIONS:

1. Preheat your oven to 400, and then get out a baking sheet. Line your baking sheet with foil before setting it to the side.
2. Get out a large bowl and toss your olive oil, rosemary, potatoes, paprika, garlic powder, sea salt, and pepper.
3. Spread your potatoes out on the baking sheet in a single layer, and bake for thirty-five minutes. They should be tender and golden brown. Serve warm.

NUTRITION: Calories: 225 Protein: 5 Grams Fat: 7 Grams Carbs: 37 Grams

48. Scalloped Tomatoes

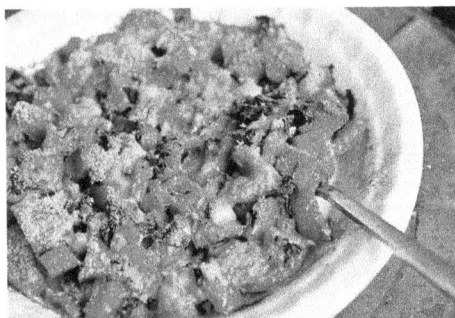

Preparation time: 10 minutes
Cooking Time: 55 Minutes
Serves: 4
INGREDIENTS:
- 1 Olive Oil, Divided
- 2 Slices Whole Wheat, Cut into ½ Inch Cubes
- 2 ¼ lbs. Tomatoes, Cut into Eights
- 2 Tablespoons Asiago Cheese, Shredded
- ¼ Cup Basil, Fresh & Chopped
- 1 Tablespoon Garlic, Minced
- ¼ Teaspoon Sea Salt, Fine

- ¼ Teaspoon Black Pepper **DIRECTIONS:**

1. Start by heating the oven to 350, and then get out an eight-by-eight-inch baking dish. Grease it with ½ teaspoon olive oil before setting the baking dish to the side.
2. Get out a large skillet, placing it over medium-high heat, and heating the remaining olive oil.
3. Add in your bread cubes and sauté for four minutes. They should be golden on all sides and then add in your garlic. Stir and cook for two minutes. Add in your tomatoes and cook for another two minutes.
4. Remove it from the skillet, and season with salt and pepper. Stir in your basil, and then transfer to your baking dish.
5. Sprinkle your asiago cheese on the top, and bake for a half-hour.

NUTRITION: Calories: 127 Protein: 5 Grams Fat: 6 Grams Carbs: 16 Grams

49. Brussels Sprouts & Pistachios

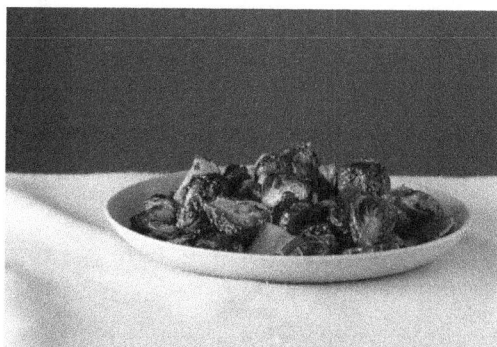

Preparation time: 6 minutes
Cooking Time: 30 Minutes
Serves: 4
INGREDIENTS:
- 1 lb. Brussels Sprouts, Trimmed & Halved Lengthwise
- 4 Shallots, Peeled & Quartered
- ½ Cup Pistachios, Roasted & Chopped
- 1/2 Lemon, Zested & Juiced
- ¼ Teaspoon Sea Salt, Fine
- ¼ Teaspoon Black Pepper
- 1 Tablespoon Olive Oil **DIRECTIONS:**

1. Preheat your oven to 400, and then get out a baking sheet. Line it with foil before placing it to the side.
2. Get out a bowl and toss your shallots and Brussels sprouts in olive oil, making sure that it's well coated.
3. Season with salt and pepper before spreading your vegetables out on the pan.
4. Bake for fifteen minutes. Your vegetables should be lightly caramelized as well as tender.
5. Until eating, remove it from the oven and toss it with lemon zest, lemon juice, and pistachios..

NUTRITION: Calories: 126 Protein: 6 Grams Fat: 7 Grams Carbs: 14 Grams

50. Mashed Celeriac

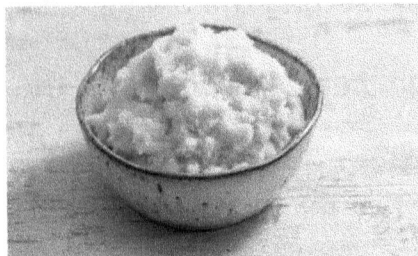

Preparation time: 5 minutes
Cooking Time: 30 Minutes
Serves: 4
INGREDIENTS:

- 2 Celery Roots, Washed, Peeled & Diced
- 1 Tablespoon Honey, Raw
- 2 Teaspoons Olive Oil
- ½ Teaspoon Nutmeg, Ground
- ¼ Teaspoon Sea Salt, Fine
- ¼ Teaspoon Black Pepper **DIRECTIONS:**

1. Preheat your oven to 400, and then get out a baking sheet. Line it with foil before setting it to the side.
2. Get out a bowl and mix your olive oil and celery root, spreading it out on the baking sheet.
3. Roast for twenty minutes. It should be lightly caramelized and tender and then place back in the bowl.
4. Add your honey and nutmeg before mashing with a potato masher—season with salt and pepper before serving.

NUTRITION: Calories: 136 Protein: 4 Grams Fat: 3 Grams Carbs: 26 Grams

51. Fennel Wild Rice

Preparation time: 5 minutes
Cooking Time: 25 Minutes
Serves: 6
INGREDIENTS:

- 1 Tablespoon Parsley, Fresh & Chopped
- 2 Cups Wild Rice, Cooked
- 1 Cup Fennel, Diced
- 1 Tablespoon Olive Oil
- ½ Cup Sweet Onion, Chopped
- ½ Red Bell Pepper, Diced Fine
- ¼ Teaspoon Sea Salt, Fine
- ¼ Teaspoon Black Pepper

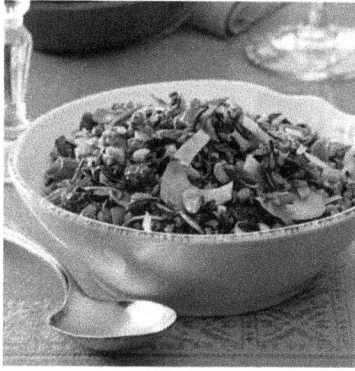

DIRECTIONS:

1. Get out a skillet and place it over medium-high heat. Heat your olive oil and add in your onion, red bell pepper, and fennel. Sauté for six minutes. It should become tender.
2. Stir in your wild rice, and cook for five minutes, and then add in your parsley—season with salt and pepper before serving warm.

NUTRITION: Calories: 222 Protein: 8 Grams Fat: 3 Grams Carbs: 43 Grams

52. Parmesan Broccoli

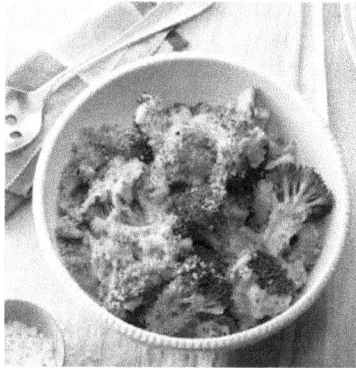

Preparation time: 3 minutes
Cooking Time: 20 Minutes
Serves: 4

INGREDIENTS:

- 2 Teaspoons Garlic, Minced
- 2 Tablespoons of Olive Oil + More for Baking Sheet Greasing
- 2 Heads Broccoli, Cut into Florets
- 1 Lemon, Zested & Juiced
- ½ Cup Parmesan Cheese, Grated
- Sea Salt to Taste **DIRECTIONS:**

1. Preheat the into 400F, and then get a baking sheet out of it. Grease with olive oil before throwing it aside.
2. Get a large bowl out and toss your broccoli with garlic, lemon zest, lemon juice, olive oil, and sea salt. Spread this mixture on the baking sheet. Make sure it's on a single layer, and then sprinkle with Parmesan cheese.
3. Bake for ten minutes. Your broccoli should be tender and then serve warm.

NUTRITION: Calories: 154 Protein: 9 Grams Fat: 11 Grams Carbs: 10 Grams

MEAT MAINS

53. Braised Beef In Oregano-tomato Sauce

Preparation time: 25 minutes
Cooking Time: 1 Hour And 30 Minutes **Servings:** 12
INGREDIENTS:

- 2 onions, chopped
- 3 celery stalks, diced
- 4 cloves garlic, minced
- 2 (28-ounce) cans of Italian-style stewed tomatoes
- 1 cup dry red wine
- 1 teaspoon dried oregano
- 1 teaspoon salt
- 3 pounds of boneless beef toast, sliced into 1-1/2-inch cubes.
- 1/2 cup chopped fresh parsley
- 1/4 cup vegetable oil
- 3/4 teaspoon black pepper **DIRECTIONS:**

1. Place a pot on medium-high fire and heat for 2 minutes.
2. Add oil and heat for another 2 minutes.
3. Add beef and brown on all sides—around 12 minutes.
4. Add the onions, celery, and garlic, and sauté for five minutes or until the vegetables are tender. Attach the remaining ingredients and bring them to a boil..
5. Reduce heat to low, cover, and simmer for 60 minutes or until beef is forktender.

NUTRITION: Calories 285 Carbs: 7.4g Protein: 31.7g Fats: 14.6g

54. Pork Chops and Herbed Tomato Sauce

Preparation time: 2 minutes
Cooking Time: 10 Minutes
Servings: 4
INGREDIENTS:

- 4 pork loin chops, boneless
- 6 tomatoes, peeled and crushed
- 3 tablespoons parsley, chopped
- 2 tablespoons olive oil
- ¼ cup kalamata olives pitted and halved
- 1 yellow onion, chopped
- 1 garlic clove, minced **DIRECTIONS:**

1. Over medium heat, heat a pan with the oil, add the pork chops, cook on each side for 3 minutes, and divide between plates.
2. Heat the same pan again over medium heat, add the tomatoes, parsley, and the rest of the ingredients, whisk, simmer for 4 minutes, drizzle over the chops and serve.

NUTRITION: Calories 334 Fat 17 Fiber 2 Carbs 12 Protein 34

55. Pita Chicken Burger with Spicy Yogurt

Preparation time: 3 minutes
Cooking Time: 15 Minutes
Servings: 4
INGREDIENTS:
- ½ cup chopped green onions
- ½ cup diced tomato
- ½ cup plain low-fat yogurt
- ½ tsp coarsely ground black pepper
- 1 ½ tsp. chopped fresh oregano
- 1 lb. ground chicken
- 1 tbsp. olive oil
- 1 tbsp. Greek or Moroccan seasoning blend
- 1/3 cup Italian seasoned breadcrumbs
- 2 cups shredded lettuce
- 2 large egg whites, lightly beaten
- 2 tsps. grated lemon rind, divided
- 4 pcs of 6-inch pitas, cut in half

DIRECTIONS:
1. Mix the ground chicken, 1 tsp thoroughly. Lemon rind, egg whites, black pepper, Greek or Moroccan seasoning, and green onions. Equally, separate into eight parts and shape each portion into ¼ inch thick patty.
2. Put fire on medium-high and place a large skillet. Fry the patties until browned or for two mins each side. Then slow the fire to medium, cover the skillet and continue cooking for another four minutes.
3. In a small bowl, mix the oregano, yogurt, and 1 tsp—lemon rind thoroughly.
4. To serve, spread the mixture on the pita, add cooked patty, 1 tbsp: Tomato, and ¼ cup lettuce.

NUTRITION: Calories: 434.3 Carbs: 44g Protein: 30.6g Fat: 15.1g

56. Beef Brisket and Veggies

Preparation time: 15 minutes
Cooking Time: 4 Hours
Servings: 10
INGREDIENTS:

- 3-pound beef brisket
- 1 carrot, peeled, chopped
- 1 onion, peeled
- 1 garlic clove, peeled
- 1 teaspoon peppercorns
- 1 teaspoon salt
- 1 teaspoon ground black pepper
- 1 bay leaf
- ½ cup crushed tomatoes
- 3 cups of water
- 1 celery stalk, chopped **DIRECTIONS:**

1. Place the beef brisket in the saucepan.
2. Add carrot, onion, garlic clove, peppercorns, salt, ground black pepper, bay leaf, crushed tomatoes, celery stalk, and water.
3. Secure the lid and bring it to a boil with the meat.
4. Simmer the meat for 4 hours over medium heat.
5. Serve the poached meat vegetables.

NUTRITION: Calories 321 Fat 10.5 Fiber 0.9 Carbs 3 Protein 50.4

57. Stewed Chicken Greek Style

Preparation time: 10 minutes
Cooking Time: 1 Hour And 15 Minutes **Servings:** 10

INGREDIENTS:
- ½ cup red wine
- 1 ½ cups chicken stock or more if needed
- 1 cup olive oil
- 1 cup tomato sauce
- 1 pc, 4lbs whole chicken cut into pieces
- 1 pinch dried oregano or to taste
- 10 small shallots, peeled
- 2 bay leaves
- 2 cloves garlic, finely chopped
- 2 tbsp. chopped fresh parsley
- 2 tsp. butter
- Salt and ground black pepper to taste **DIRECTIONS:**

1. Bring to a boil a large pot of lightly salted water. Mix in the shallots and let boil uncovered until tender for around three minutes. Then drain the shallots and dip in cold water until no longer warm.
2. In another large pot over medium fire, heat butter and olive oil until bubbling and melted. Then sauté in the chicken and shallots for 15 minutes or until chicken is cooked and shallots are soft and translucent.

3. Add the chopped garlic and cook for an additional three minutes.
4. Then add bay leaves, oregano, salt and pepper, parsley, tomato sauce, and the red wine and let simmer for a minute before adding the chicken stock. Stir before covering and let cook for 50 minutes on medium-low fire or until chicken is tender.

NUTRITION: Calories: 644.8 Carbs: 8.2g Protein: 62.1g Fat: 40.4g

58. Hot Pork Meatballs

Preparation time: 2 minutes
Cooking Time: 10 Minutes
Servings: 2
INGREDIENTS:
- 4 oz. pork loin, grinded
- ½ teaspoon garlic powder
- ¼ teaspoon chili powder
- ¼ teaspoon cayenne pepper
- ¼ teaspoon ground black pepper
- ¼ teaspoon white pepper
- 1 tablespoon water
- 1 teaspoon olive oil   **DIRECTIONS:**

1. Mix up together ground meat, garlic powder, cayenne pepper, ground black pepper, white pepper, and water.
2. With the help of the fingertips, make the small meatballs.
3. Heat olive oil in the skillet.
4. Arrange the kite in the oil and cook them for 10 minutes. Flip the kofte on another side from time to time.

NUTRITION: Calories 162 Fat 10.3 Fiber 0.3 Carbs 1 Protein 15.7

59. Beef and Zucchini Skillet

Preparation time: 10 minutes
Cooking Time: 20 Minutes
Servings: 2

INGREDIENTS:
- 2 oz. ground beef
- ½ onion, sliced
- ½ bell pepper, sliced
- 1 tablespoon butter
- ½ teaspoon salt
- 1 tablespoon tomato sauce
- 1 small zucchini, chopped
- ½ teaspoon dried oregano   **DIRECTIONS:**

1. Place the ground beef in the skillet.
2. Add salt, butter, and dried oregano.
3. Mix up the meat mixture and cook it for 10 minutes.
4. After this, transfer the cooked ground beef to the bowl.
5. Place zucchini, bell pepper, and onion in the skillet (where the ground meat was cooking) and roast the vegetables for 7 minutes over medium heat or tender.
6. Then add cooked ground beef and tomato sauce. Mix up well.
7. Cook the beef toss for 2-3 minutes over medium heat.

NUTRITION: Calories 182 Fat 8.7 Fiber 0.1 Carbs 0.3 Protein 24.1

SEAFOOD MAINS

60. Mussels with tomatoes & chili

Preparation time: 7 minutes
Cooking time: 20 minutes
Servings: 4
INGREDIENTS

- 2 ripe tomatoes
- 2 tbsps. olive oil
- 1 tsp. tomato paste
- 1 garlic clove, chopped
- 1 shallot, chopped
- 1 chopped red or green chili
- A small glass of dry white wine
- Salt and pepper to taste
- 2 lbs./900 g. mussels, cleaned
- Basil leaves, fresh

DIRECTIONS:

1. Add tomatoes to boiling water for 3 minutes, then drain.
2. Peel the tomatoes and chop the flesh.
3. Add oil to an iron skillet and heat to sauté shallots and garlic for 3 minutes.
4. Stir in wine along with tomatoes, chili, and salt/pepper, and tomato paste.
5. Cook for 2 minutes, then add mussels.
6. Cover and after thatn let it steam for 4 minutes.
7. Garnish with basil leaves and serve warm.

NUTRITION: Calories 483 total fat 15.2 g Sat. fat 2.4 g Carbs 20.4 g Fiber 1.9 g Sugars 7.3 g Protein 62.3 g Sodium 890 mg

61. Lemon Garlic Shrimp

Preparation time: 6 minutes
Cooking time: 25 minutes
Servings: 6
INGREDIENTS

- 4 tsps. extra-virgin olive oil, divided
- 2 red bell peppers, diced
- 2 lbs./900 g. fresh asparagus, sliced
- 2 tsps. lemon zest, freshly grated
- ½ tsp. salt, divided
- 5 garlic cloves, minced
- 1 lb./450 g. peeled raw shrimp, deveined

- 1 c. reduced-sodium chicken broth or water
- 1 tsp. cornstarch
- 2 tbsps. lemon juice
- 2 tbsps. fresh parsley, chopped **DIRECTIONS:**

1. Add 2 teaspoon oil to a large skillet and heat for a minute.
2. Stir in asparagus, lemon zest, bell pepper, and salt. Sauté for 6 minutes.
3. Keep the sautéed veggies in a separate bowl.
4. Add remaining oil to the same pan and add garlic.
5. Sauté for 30 seconds, then add shrimp—Cook for 1 min.
6. Mix cornstarch with broth in a bowl and pour this mixture into the pan.
7. Add salt and stir cook for 2 minutes.
8. Turn off the flame, then add parsley and lemon juice.
9. Serve warm with sautéed vegetables.

NUTRITION: Calories 204 total fat 4 g Sat. fat 0.9 g Carbs 23.6 g Fiber 1.2 g Sugars 1.7 g Protein 17. 1 g Sodium 522 mg

62. Pepper Tilapia with Spinach

Preparation time: 5 minutes
Cooking:time:30minutes
Servings: 6
INGREDIENTS

- 4 tilapia fillets, 8 oz./ 227 g. each
- 4 c. fresh spinach
- 1 red onion, sliced
- 3 garlic cloves, minced
- 2 tbsps. extra virgin olive oil
- 3 lemons
- 1 tbsp. ground black pepper
- 1 tbsp. ground white pepper
- 1 tbsp. crushed red pepper **DIRECTIONS:**

1. Preheat at 350°F/176.6°C.
2. Place the fish in a small baking dish with two lemon juices.
3. Cover the fish in the lemon juice and then sprinkle the three types of pepper over the fish.
4. Slice the remaining lemon and cover the fish—Bake in the oven for 20 minutes.
5. While the fish cooks, sauté the garlic and onion in the olive oil. Add the spinach and sauté for 7 more minutes.
6. Top the fish with spinach and serve.

NUTRITION: Calories 323 total fat 11.4 g Sat. fat 2.2 g Carbs 10.4 g Fiber 2.7 g Sugar 1.3 g Protein 50 g Sodium 145 mg

63. Spicy Shrimp Salad

Preparation time: 5 minutes
Cooking time: 5 minutes
Servings: 2
INGREDIENTS

- ½ lb./225 g. salad shrimp, chopped
- 2 stalks celery, chopped
- ¼ c. red onion, diced
- 1 tsp. black pepper • 1 tsp. red pepper
- 1 tbsp. lemon juice
- Dash of cayenne pepper
- 1 tbsp. olive oil
- 2 cucumbers, sliced

METHOD

1. Combine the shrimp, celery, and onion in a bowl and mix.
2. In a separate bowl, whisk the oil and the lemon juice, add red pepper, black pepper, and cayenne pepper. Pour over the shrimp and mix.
3. Serve with slices of thickly cut cucumber on it and enjoy.

NUTRITION: Calories: 245 Total fat: 9g Sat Fat: 1.2g Carbs: 18.2g Fiber: 3.2g Sugar: 9g Protein: 27.3g Sodium: 280 mg

64. Baked Cod in Parchment

Preparation time: 5 minutes
Cooking time: 30 minutes
Servings: 1
INGREDIENTS

- 1-2 potatoes, sliced
- 5 cherry tomatoes, halved
- 5 pitted olives
- Juice of ½ lemon
- ½ tbsp. olive oil
- 4 oz./115 g. cod
- 20 inches long parchment
- Sea salt and black pepper **DIRECTIONS:**

1. Preheat at 350°F/176.6°C.
2. Spread the olive oil on parchment and arrange potato on it.
3. In a separate bowl, combine the tomatoes, olives, and lemon juice.
4. Put the fish fillet on potatoes and top with tomato mixture.
5. Add salt and pepper.
6. Fold the filled parchment squares and bake for 20 minutes.

NUTRITION: Calories 330 total fat 8 g Sat. fat 1 g Carbs 35 g Fiber 5 g Sugars 7 g Protein 25 g Sodium 350 mg

65. Thai Tuna Bowl

Preparation time: 6 minutes
Cooking time: 10 minutes
Servings: 1
INGREDIENTS

- ½ c. cooked quinoa, at room temperature
- ½ c. spiraled zucchini
- 1 carrot, spiraled
- ¼ c. chopped red cabbage
- 2 tbsps. Diced red onion
- ¼ c. roasted chickpeas
- oz./156 g. White Albacore Tuna, drained
- Cilantro
- Juice of 1 lime
- Simple Thai Peanut Dressing   **DIRECTIONS:**
1. Add quinoa to the bottom of a large bowl.
2. Add zucchini noodles, cabbage, onion, chickpeas, tuna, and carrot to the bowl.
3. Top with cilantro and lime juice.
4. Stir in a peanut dressing and serve.

NUTRITION: Calories 246 Total fat 7.4 g Sat. fat 3.1 g Carbs 15.3 g Fiber 8.8 g Sugars 11.6 g Protein 12.4gSodium 1054 mg

66. Roasted Fish & New Potatoes

Preparation time: 10 minutes
Cooking time: 35 minutes
Servings: 4
INGREDIENTS

- 3 tbsps. extra-virgin olive oil
- 3 tbsps. orange juice
- 3 tbsps. white vinegar
- ½ tsp. orange peel, grated
- ¼ tsp. dried dill weed
- 12 new potatoes, cubed
- 4 salmon fillets, skin removed   **DIRECTIONS:**
1. Preheat oven to 420°F/215°C.
2. Blend the first five ingredients.
3. Sprinkle potato with 2 tbsps. Of this mixture. Bake for 20 minutes.
4. Sprinkle fillets with the remaining mixture and add to the potatoes.

5. Cook for about 15 min and serve.
NUTRITION: Calories 289 total fat 8.2 g Sat. fat 1.3 g Carbs 23.4 g Fiber 2.2 g Sugars 2 g Protein 29 g Sodium 430 mg

POULTRY MAINS

67. Turkey Burgers with Mango Salsa

Preparation time: 15 minutes
Cooking time: 10 minutes
Servings: 6
INGREDIENTS:

- 1½ pounds ground turkey breast
- 1 teaspoon sea salt, divided
- ¼ teaspoon freshly ground black pepper
- 2 tablespoons extra-virgin olive oil
- 2 mangos, peeled, pitted, and cubed
- ½ red onion, finely chopped
- Juice of 1 lime
- 1 garlic clove, minced
- ½ jalapeño pepper, seeded and finely minced
- 2 tablespoons chopped fresh cilantro leaves **DIRECTIONS:**

1. Form the turkey breast into 4 patties and season with ½ teaspoon of sea salt and pepper.
2. Heat the olive oil until it shimmers in a large nonstick skillet over mediumhigh heat.
3. Add the turkey patties and cook for about 5 minutes per side until browned.
4. While the patties cook, mix the mango, red onion, lime juice, garlic, jalapeño, cilantro, and remaining ½ teaspoon of sea salt in a small bowl. Spoon the salsa over the turkey patties and serve.

VARIATION TIP: Serve this salsa over grilled halibut. Heat the grill to medium-high heat and brush it with olive oil. Grill 4 (4- to 6-ounce) halibut fillets for about 6 minutes per side. Top with the salsa.
NUTRITION: Calories: 384g Protein: 34g Total Carbohydrates: 27g Sugars: 24g; Fiber: 3g Total Fat: 16g Saturated Fat: 3g Cholesterol: 84mg Sodium: 543mg

68. Herb-Roasted Turkey Breast

Preparation time: 15 minutes
Cooking time: 1½ hours (plus 20 minutes to rest) **Serves**
6
INGREDIENTS:

- 2 tablespoons extra-virgin olive oil
- 4 garlic cloves, minced
- Zest of 1 lemon
- 1 tablespoon chopped fresh thyme leaves
- 1 tablespoon chopped fresh rosemary leaves
- 2 tablespoons chopped fresh Italian parsley leaves
- 1 teaspoon ground mustard
- 1 teaspoon sea salt
- ¼ teaspoon freshly ground black pepper
- 1 (6-pound) bone-in, skin-on turkey breast
- 1 cup dry white wine **DIRECTIONS:**

1. Preheat the oven to 325°F.
2. Place the olive oil, garlic, lemon zest, thyme, rosemary, parsley, mustard, sea salt, and pepper in a small cup.
3. Put the herb mixture evenly over the turkey breast's surface, loosen the skin, and rub underneath as well. Place the turkey breast in a roasting pan on a rack, skin-side up
4. Pour the wine into the pan. Roast for 1 to 1½ hours until the turkey reaches an internal temperature of 165°F. In a shallow cup, whisk together the olive oil, garlic, lemon zest, thyme, rosemary, parsley, mustard, sea salt, and pepper..

MAKE IT A MEAL: Serve alongside Sweet Potato Mash (here) and Easy Brussels Sprouts Hash (here) for a complete meal.

NUTRITION: Calories: 392 Protein: 84g Total Carbohydrates: 2g Sugars: <1g Fiber: <1g Total Fat: 6g Saturated Fat: <1g Cholesterol: 210m Sodium: 479mg

69. Chicken Sausage and Peppers

Preparation time: 10 minutes
Cooking time: 20 minutes
Serves 6
INGREDIENTS:
- 2 tablespoons extra-virgin olive oil
- 6 Italian chicken sausage links
- 1 onion
- 1 red bell pepper
- 1 green bell pepper
- 3 garlic cloves, minced
- ½ cup dry white wine
- ½ teaspoon sea salt
- ¼ teaspoon freshly ground black pepper **DIRECTIONS:**

1. Pinch red pepper flakes
2. Heat the olive oil until it shines in a large skillet over medium-high heat

3. Add the sausages and cook for 5 to 7 minutes, occasionally turning, until browned, and they reach an internal temperature of 165°F. With tongs, remove the link from the pan and set it aside on a platter, tented with aluminum foil to keep warm.

4. Return the skillet to heat and add the onion, red bell pepper, and green bell pepper. Cook, stirring regularly, for 5 to 7 minutes, until the vegetables begin to brown.

5. Add the garlic and simmer for 30 seconds, stirring continuously.

6. Stir in the wine, sea salt, pepper, and red pepper flakes. Using the spoon to scrape and fold in some browned fragments from the bottom of the plate. Simmer for about 4 minutes, stirring until the liquid decreases by half. Spoon the peppers over the sausages and serve.

SUBSTITUTION TIP: For a different flavor profile, add one fennel bulb, thinly shaved, in place of the green bell peppers—Cook as directed in the recipe.

NUTRITION: Calories: 173 Protein: 22g Total Carbohydrates: 6g Sugars: 2g Fiber: <1g Total Fat: 5g Saturated Fat: 1g Cholesterol: 85mg Sodium: 1,199mg

70. Chicken Piccata

Preparation time: 10 minutes
Cooking time: 15 minutes
Serves 6
INGREDIENTS:
- ½ cup whole-wheat flour
- ½ teaspoon sea salt
- 1/8 teaspoon freshly ground black pepper
- 11/2 pounds of boneless, skinless chicken breasts, sliced into 6 pieces and pounded 1/2 inch thick (see tip)
- 3 tablespoons extra-virgin olive oil
- 1 cup unsalted chicken broth
- ½ cup dry white wine
- Juice of 1 lemon
- Zest of 1 lemon
- ¼ cup capers drained and rinsed
- ¼ cup chopped fresh parsley leaves **DIRECTIONS:**

1. In a shallow dish, whisk the flour, sea salt, and pepper. Dredge the chicken in the flour and tap off any excess.

2. Heat the olive oil until it shimmers in a large skillet over medium-high heat.

3. Add the chicken and cook for about 4 minutes per side until browned. To preserve temperature, remove the chicken from the pan and set aside, tented with aluminum foil.

4. Return the skillet to heat and add the broth, wine, lemon juice, lemon zest, and capers. Use the side of a spoon to scrape and fold in any browned bits from the pan's bottom. Simmer for 3 to 4 minutes, stirring, until the liquid thickens.

Remove the skillet from the heat and return the chicken to the pan. Turn to coat. Stir in the parsley and serve.

COOKING TIP: To pound the chicken to an even thickness: Place the chicken between two pieces of plastic wrap or parchment paper and use a flat kitchen mallet or a smooth-bottomed heavy saucepan to pound until they reach the desired thickness. Use caution to avoid puncturing the plastic or paper.

NUTRITION: Calories: 153 Protein: 8g Total Carbohydrates: 9g Sugars: <1g Fiber: <1g Total Fat: 9g Saturated Fat: 1g Cholesterol: 19mg Sodium: 352mg

71. One-Pan Tuscan Chicken

Preparation time: 10 minutes
Cooking time: 25 minutes
Serves 6
INGREDIENTS:

- ¼ cup extra-virgin olive oil, divided
- Skinless chicken breasts, 1 pound boneless, sliced into 3/4-inch sections
- 1 onion, chopped
- 1 red bell pepper, chopped
- 3 garlic cloves, minced
- ½ cup dry white wine
- 1 (14-ounce) can crushed tomatoes, untrained
- 1 (14-ounce) can chopped tomatoes, drained
- 1 (14-ounce) can white beans, drained
- 1 tablespoon dried Italian seasoning
- ½ teaspoon sea salt
- 1/8 teaspoon freshly ground black pepper
- 1/8 teaspoon red pepper flakes
- ¼ cup chopped fresh basil leaves **DIRECTIONS:**

1. Over medium-high pressure, heat 2 teaspoons of olive oil in a large skillet until it shimmers.
2. Add the chicken and cook for about 6 minutes, stirring, until browned. Remove the chicken from the skillet and set it aside on a platter, tented with aluminum foil to keep warm.
3. Return the skillet to heat and heat the remaining 2 tablespoons of olive oil until it shimmers.
4. Add the onion and red bell pepper. Cook for about 5 minutes, occasionally stirring, until the vegetables are soft.
5. Attach the garlic and fry, stirring continuously, for 30 seconds.
6. Stir in the wine, and use the spoon's side to scrape and fold in any browned bits from the bottom of the pan. Cook for 1 minute, stirring.
7. Add the crushed and chopped tomatoes, white beans, Italian seasoning, sea salt, pepper, and red pepper flakes. Bring it to a boil and bring the heat down to medium. Cook for 5 minutes, sometimes stirring.

8. Return to the skillet the chicken and any juices that have accumulated. Simmer for 1 to 2 minutes before the chicken heats up. Remove from the heat and before eating, mix in the basil.

VARIATION TIP: Add ½ cup chopped black or green olives and 1 cup thawed frozen spinach when you return the chicken to the pan. Note that the fat content will increase.

NUTRITION: Per Serving Calories: 271 Protein: 14g Total Carbohydrates: 29g Sugars: 8g Fiber: 8g Total Fat: 0g Saturated Fat: 1g Cholesterol: 14mg Sodium: 306mg

72. Chicken Kapama

Preparation time: 10 minutes
Cooking time: 2 hours
Serves 4
INGREDIENTS:
- 1 (32-ounce) can chopped tomatoes, drained
- ¼ cup dry white wine
- 2 tablespoons tomato paste
- 3 tablespoons extra-virgin olive oil
- ¼ teaspoon red pepper flakes
- 1 teaspoon ground allspice
- ½ teaspoon dried oregano
- 2 whole cloves
- 1 cinnamon stick
- ½ teaspoon sea salt
- 1/8 teaspoon freshly ground black pepper
- 4 boneless, skinless chicken breast halves **DIRECTIONS:**

1. Combine the tomatoes, wine, tomato paste, olive oil, red pepper flakes, allspice, oregano, garlic, cinnamon stick, sea salt and pepper in a big pot over medium-high heat. Bring to a boil, sometimes stirring.
2. Set the heat to medium-low and boil, stirring periodically for 30 minutes. Remove all the cloves and cinnamon sticks from the sauce and let the sauce cool.
3. Preheat the oven to 350°F.
4. Place the chicken in a 9-by-13-inch baking dish. Pour the sauce over the chicken and cover the pan with aluminum foil—Bake for 40 to 45 minutes, or until the chicken reaches an internal temperature of 165°F.

MAKE IT A MEAL: Serve this dish spooned over ¾ cup (per serving) cooked wholewheat pasta.

NUTRITION: 220; Protein: 8g Total Carbohydrates: 11g Sugars: 7g; Fiber: 3g Total Fat: 14g Saturated Fat: 3g Cholesterol: 19mg Sodium: 273mg

73. Spinach and Feta–Stuffed Chicken Breasts

Preparation time: 10 minutes
Cooking time: 45 minutes
Servings: 4
INGREDIENTS:

- 2 tablespoons extra-virgin olive oil
- 1 pound fresh baby spinach
- 3 garlic cloves, minced
- Zest of 1 lemon
- ½ teaspoon sea salt
- 1/8 teaspoon freshly ground black pepper
- ½ cup crumbled feta cheese
- 4 skinless, boneless chicken breast pieces, pounded to the thickness of 1/2 inch

DIRECTIONS:

1. Preheat the oven to 350°F.
2. Heat the olive oil until it shimmers in a large skillet over medium-high heat..
3. Add the spinach. Cook for 3 to 4 minutes, stirring until wilted.
4. Add the garlic, lemon zest, sea salt, and pepper. Cook for 30 seconds, stirring constantly. Cool slightly and mix in the cheese.
5. Spread spinach cheese mixture in an even layer over the chicken pieces and roll the breast around the filling. Hold closed with toothpicks or butcher's twine. Place breasts 9-by-13-inch baking dish and bakes for 30 to 40 minutes, or until the chicken reaches an internal temperature of 165°F.
6. Serve !

COOKING TIP: If you use toothpicks to hold the chicken rolls closed, soak them in water for about 5 minutes first to prevent burning.

NUTRITION: Calories: 263; Protein: 17g; Total Carbohydrates: 7g; Sugars: 3g; Fiber: 3g; Total Fat: 20g; Saturated Fat: 9g; Cholesterol: 63mg; Sodium: 901mg

VEGETABLES MAINS

74. Peppers and Lentils Salad

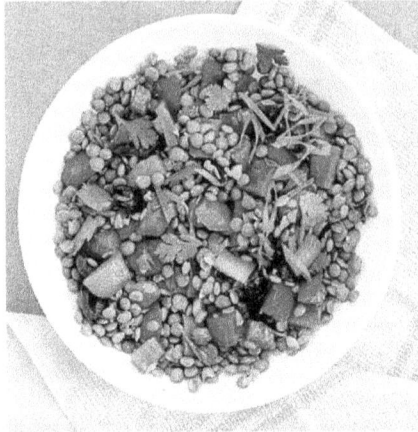

Preparation Time: 10 minutes
Cooking Time: 0 minutes
Servings: 4
INGREDIENTS:

- 14 oz. canned lentils drained and rinsed
- Two spring onions, chopped
- 1 red bell pepper, chopped
- 1 green bell pepper, chopped
- 1 tbsp. fresh lime juice
- 1/3 cup coriander, chopped
- 2 tsp. balsamic vinegar   **DIRECTIONS:**

1. In a salad bowl, combine the lentils with the onions, bell peppers, and the rest of the ingredients, toss and serve.

NUTRITION: Calories 200 Fat: 2.45g Fiber: 6.7g Carbs: 10.5g Protein: 5.6g

75. Olives and Lentils Salad

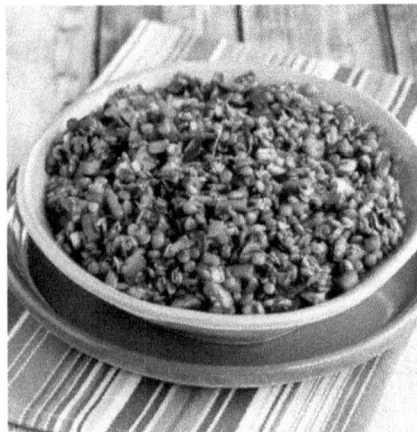

Preparation Time: 10 minutes
Cooking Time: 0 minutes
Servings: 2
INGREDIENTS:

- 1/3 cup canned green lentils, drained and rinsed
- 1 tbsp. olive oil
- 2 cups baby spinach
- 1 cup black olives, pitted and halved
- 2 tbsps. sunflower seeds
- 1 tbsp. Dijon mustard
- 2 tbsps. balsamic vinegar
- 2 tbsps. olive oil   **DIRECTIONS:**

1. In a bowl, mix the lentils with the spinach, olives, and the rest of the ingredients, toss and serve cold.

NUTRITION: Calories 279 Fat: 6.5g Fiber: 4.5g Carbs: 9.6g Protein: 12g

76. Lime Spinach and Chickpeas Salad

Preparation Time: 10 minutes
Cooking Time: 0 minutes
Servings: 4
INGREDIENTS:

- 16 oz. canned chickpeas, drained and rinsed
- 2 cups baby spinach leaves
- ½ tbsp. lime juice
- 2 tbsps. olive oil
- 1 tsp. cumin, ground
- A pinch of salt and black pepper
- ½ tsp. chili flakes   **DIRECTIONS:**

1. In a bowl, mix the chickpeas with the spinach and the rest of the ingredients, toss, and serve cold.

NUTRITION: Calories 240 Fat: 8.2g Fiber: 5.3g. Carbs: 11.6g Protein: 12g

77. Beans and Cucumber Salad

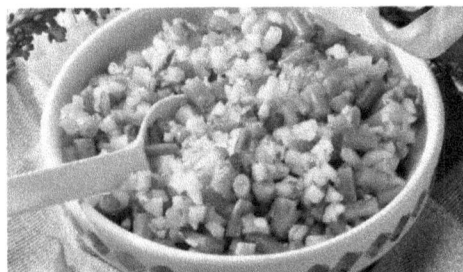

Preparation Time: 10 minutes
Cooking Time: 0 minutes
Servings: 4
INGREDIENTS:

- 15 ouz. Canned broad northern beans, drained and rinsed
- 2 tbsps. olive oil
- ½ cup baby arugula
- 1 cup cucumber, sliced
- 1 tbsp. parsley, chopped
- 2 tomatoes, cubed
- A pinch of salt and black pepper
- 2 tbsp. balsamic vinegar   **DIRECTIONS:**

1. In a cup, blend the beans with the cucumber and the rest of the ingredients, toss and eat cold.

NUTRITION: Calories 233 Fat: 9g, Fiber: 6.5g Carbs: 13g Protein: 8g

78. Tomato and Avocado Salad

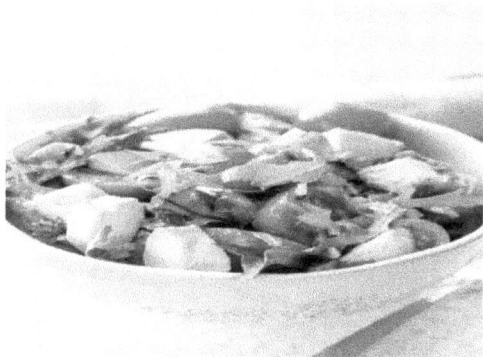

Preparation Time: 10 minutes
Cooking Time: 0 minutes
Servings: 4
INGREDIENTS:

- 1 lb. cherry tomatoes, cubed
- 2 avocados, pitted, peeled and cubed
- 1 sweet onion, chopped
- A pinch of salt and black pepper
- 2 tbsps. lemon juice
- 1 and ½ tbsps. olive oil
- A handful basil, chopped   **DIRECTIONS:**

1. In a dish, mix the tomatoes with the avocados and the rest of the ingredients, stir and serve immediately.

NUTRITION: Calories 148 Fat: 7.8g Fiber: 2.9g Carbs: 5.4g Protein: 5.5g

79. Corn and Tomato Salad

Preparation Time: 10 minutes
Cooking Time: 0 minutes
Servings: 4
INGREDIENTS:

- 2 avocados, pitted, peeled and cubed   • 1 pint of mixed cherry tomatoes, halved:
- 2 tbsps. avocado oil
- 1 tbsp. lime juice
- ½ tsp. lime zest, grated
- A pinch of salt and black pepper
- ¼ cup dill, chopped   **DIRECTIONS:**

1. In a salad bowl, mix the avocados with the tomatoes and the rest of the ingredients, toss, and serve cold.

NUTRITION: Calories 188 Fat: 7.3g Fiber: 4.9g Carbs: 6.4gProtein: 6.5g

80. Orange and Cucumber Salad

Preparation Time: 10 minutes
Cooking Time: 0 minutes
Servings: 4
INGREDIENTS:

- 2 cucumbers, sliced
- 1 orange, peeled and cut into segments
- 1 cup cherry tomatoes, halved
- 1 small red onion, chopped
- 3 tbsps. olive oil
- 4 ½ tsps. balsamic vinegar
- Salt and black pepper to the taste
- 1 tbsp. lemon juice **DIRECTIONS:**

1. In a dish, blend the cucumbers with the orange and the rest of the ingredients, toss and eat.

NUTRITION: Calories 102 Fat: 7.5g Fiber: 3g Carbs: 6.1g Protein: 3.4g

81. Parsley and Corn Salad

Preparation Time: 10 minutes
Cooking Time: 0 minutes
Servings: 4
INGREDIENTS:

- 1 ½ tsps. balsamic vinegar
- 2 tbsps. lime juice
- 2 tbsps. olive oil
- A pinch of salt and black pepper
- Black pepper to the taste
- 4 cups corn
- ½ cup parsley, chopped
- 2 spring onions, chopped **DIRECTIONS:**

1. In a salad bowl, combine the corn with the onions and the rest of the ingredients, toss, and serve cold.

NUTRITION: Calories 121 Fat: 9.5g Fiber: 1.8g Carbs: 4.1g Protein: 1.9g

82. Lettuce and Onions Salad

Preparation Time: 10 minutes
Cooking Time: 0 minutes
Servings: 4
INGREDIENTS:

- ¼ cup lime juice
- 1 garlic clove, minced

- Salt and black pepper to the taste
- 2 tbsps. olive oil
- 1 green head lettuce, chopped
- 2 red onions, chopped
- 4 tomatoes, chopped
- ½ cup cilantro, chopped **DIRECTIONS:**

1. In a bowl, mix the lettuce with the onions and the rest of the ingredients, toss, and serve right away.

NUTRITION: Calories 103 Fat: 3g Fiber: 2g Carbs: 3g Protein: 2g

83. Sweet Potato and Eggplant Mix

Preparation Time: 10 minutes
Cooking Time: 15 minutes
Servings: 4
INGREDIENTS:

- 2 baby eggplants, cubed
- 2 sweet potatoes, cubed
- 1 tbsp. olive oil
- 1 red onion, cut into wedges
- 1 tsp. hot paprika
- 2 tsp. cumin, ground
- Salt and black pepper to the taste
- 4 cups baby spinach
- ¼ cup lime juice **DIRECTIONS:**

1. Heat a pan with the oil over medium-high heat, add the eggplants and the potatoes and sauté for 5 minutes.
2. Add the remaining ingredients, minus spinach, toss and simmer for another 10 minutes..
3. Add the spinach, toss, divide into bowls and serve.

NUTRITION: Calories 200 Fat: 8.3g Fiber: 3.4g Carbs: 12.4g Protein: 4.5g

84. Tomato and Beans Salad

Preparation Time: 10 minutes
Cooking Time: 0 minutes
Servings: 4
INGREDIENTS:

- 2 tomatoes, cubed
- 2 cups of canned black beans, washed and drained.
- 1 garlic clove, minced
- 1 yellow onion, chopped
- 1 tbsp. olive oil
- Salt and black pepper to the taste

- ¼ tsp. cumin, ground **DIRECTIONS:**

1. In a dish, mix the tomatoes with the beans and the other ingredients, stir and eat.

NUTRITION: Calories 200 Fat: 8.7g Fiber: 3.4g Carbs: 6.5g Protein: 5.4g

BEANS, RICE, AND GRAINS

85. Chickpea and Rice

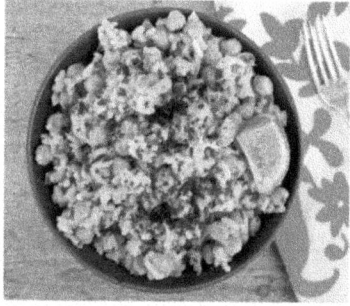

Preparation Time: 30 min.
Cooking Time: 45 min.
Servings: 4
INGREDIENTS:

- 0.3 lb. long - grain rice, soaked in water for 20 minutes
- 0.3 lb. chickpeas, cooked
- Salt and pepper, to taste
- 1 bay leaf
- 2 tablespoons chopped parsley
- 1 garlic clove minced
- .4 quarts of chicken broth
- 3 tablespoons olive oil
- 1 medium onion, sliced
- 1 teaspoon lime juice **DIRECTIONS:**

1. Drain the rice and set aside.
2. Heat oil in saucepan and cook onion with garlic until onion is softened.
3. Add chickpeas, bay leaf, salt, and pepper. Stir fry for 1-2 minutes.
4. Add chicken broth and let it simmer on medium heat until bubbles appear at the surface.
5. Add rice and lime juice and stir well. Simmer for 4-5 minutes or before the bubbles emerge on the surface or the rice. Now cover the saucepans with a lid and let rice cook on low flame for 20 minutes.
6. Add to serving dish and top with parsley.
7. Serve and enjoy!

NUTRITION: Calories – 321 Fat –17 g Carbs – 35 g Protein – 21 g

86. One-Pot Rice and Chicken

Preparation Time: 30 min.
Cooking Time: 45 min.

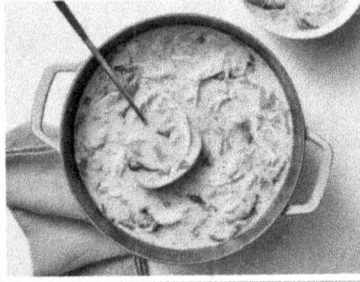

Servings: 4

INGREDIENTS:

- 4-5 chicken thighs
- 0.3 lb. long - grain rice, soaked in water for 20 minutes
- ¼ teaspoons cumin seeds
- 1 teaspoon dried oregano
- Salt and pepper, to taste
- 1 garlic clove, minced
- 0.4 quarts of water
- 3 tablespoons olive oil
- 1 medium onion, sliced
- 1 teaspoon lime juice
- 1 tablespoon vinegar **DIRECTIONS:**

1. In a bowl add chicken, some salt, some black pepper, oregano, cumin, and vinegar. Mix well. Let it marinate for about 20 minutes.
2. Heat some of the oil in the pan and put chicken in the pan.. Let the chicken cook for about 5-6 minutes per side or until nicely golden from both sides. Keep turning the chicken over after a few minutes.
3. Drain the rice and set aside.
4. Preheat oven to 355° F.
5. In a pan, heat some olive oil and cook the onion with garlic until the onion has softened..
6. Add salt and pepper. Stir fry for 1-2 minutes.
7. Add water and let it simmer on medium heat until bubbles appear at the surface.
8. Add rice and lime juice and stir well. Let it simmer for 6-10 minutes or until bubbles appear at the surface or the rice and liquid are dried a little. Place chicken on top of rice.
9. Cover the skillet with a lid and place it in the oven. Bake for 20 minutes.
10. Serve and enjoy!

NUTRITION: Calories – 240 Fat, – 15 g Carbs – 3 g Protein – ½ g

87. Grain Bowl with Lentil and Chickpeas

Preparation time: 10 min.

Cooking Time: 5-8 min.
Servings: 3-4
INGREDIENTS:

- 6 tablespoons virgin olive oil
- Salt, to taste
- 1 zucchini squash, sliced into rounds
- 0.6 lb. farro, cooked
- 0.5 lb. cooked brown lentils, cooked
- ½ lb. chickpeas, cooked
- 0.3 lb. cherry tomatoes, halved
- 2 shallots, sliced
- 2 avocados, peeled, pitted and sliced
- 0.3 lb. fresh parsley, chopped
- 5-6 Kalamata olives
- 2 tablespoons lemon juice
- Some crumbled feta cheese, optional
- 2 tablespoons Dijon mustard
- 1-2 garlic cloves, minced
- 1 teaspoon sumac, ground
- Mixed spices, of choice

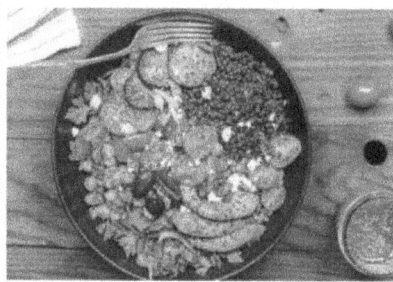

DIRECTIONS:

1. Heat 1-2 tablespoons oil in a pan and sauté zucchini until tender. Removed from heat and set aside.
2. In a bowl add Dijon mustard, some salt, sumac powder, mix spices, remaining olive oil, garlic, and lemon juice; mix well and set aside.
3. Add zucchini, avocado, shallots, farro, lentils, tomatoes, chickpeas, olives, feta, and parsley into serving bowls. Season with Dijon mustard dressing.
4. Serve and enjoy.

NUTRITION: Calories – 625 Fat, – 45 g Carbs – 0 g Protein – 15 g

88. White Beans with Vegetables

Preparation Time: 10 min.
Cooking Time: 0 min.
Servings: 4
INGREDIENTS:

- ½ lb. white beans, cooked
- 1 onion, chopped
- 1 tablespoon lemon juice
- 7-8 cherry tomatoes, chopped
- 1 tablespoon oregano
- Ground pepper, to taste
- 2-3 tablespoons cilantro, chopped
- Salt, to taste

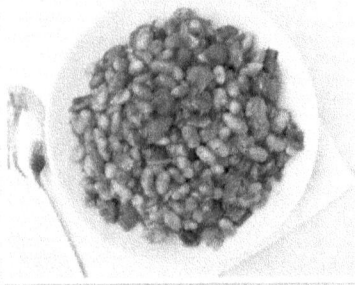

DIRECTIONS:
1. In a large bowl combine white beans, onion, tomatoes, cilantro, oregano, salt, pepper, and lemon juice.
2. Add mixture to a serving dish.
3. Enjoy.

NUTRITION: Calories – 345 Fat –27 g Carbs 67 g Protein – 21 g

89. Greek Wheat Berry Salad with Feta

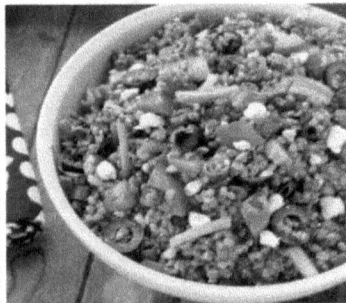

Preparation Time: 10 min.
Cooking Time: 0 min. **Servings:** 1

INGREDIENTS:
- 0.6 lb. wheat berries, cooked
- 0.2 lb. spring onion, chopped
- A handful of black olives, chopped
- 2-3 roasted red bell peppers, chopped
- 3-4 tomatoes, chopped
- 1-2 onions, sliced
- 0.3 lb. feta cheese, crumbled

- 2 chilies, sliced
- 2 tablespoons honey
- 1 teaspoon lemon juice
- Salt, to taste
- ¼ tablespoons black pepper
- 2 tablespoons olive oil
- 2 tablespoons thyme
- 4-5 tablespoons balsamic vinegar
- 1 tablespoon Dijon mustard • 4 tablespoons olive oil o lb. parsley, chopped **DIRECTIONS:**

1. In a bowl combine honey, mustard, bell peppers, salt, pepper, vinegar, olive oil. Mix well and set aside.
2. In a mixing bowl add wheat berries, thyme, onion, tomato, spring onion, parsley, chilies, and olive. Mix well.
3. Drizzle dressing on salad, add feta cheese, and mix everything.
4. Serve and enjoy.

NUTRITION: Calories – 354 Fat –29 g Carbs – 10 g Protein – 7.2 g

90. Skillet Black-Eyed Pease and Spinach

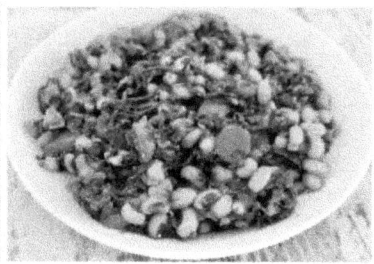

Preparation Time: 10min.
Cooking Time: 35 min.
Serving: 3-4
INGREDIENTS:
- ½ lb. dry black-eyed peas, cooked
- 4 tablespoons extra virgin olive oil
- 1 onion, chopped
- 1 carrot, sliced
- 1 red bell pepper, chopped
- 1 lb. fresh spinach, washed
- 0.2 lb. tomatoes, crushed
- ½ tablespoons fine salt
- Lemon for serving
- Ground black pepper, to taste
- 1 tablespoon fresh parsley chopped
- 0.3 quarts chicken broth **DIRECTIONS:**

1. Heat oil in a skillet and cook onion with carrots for about 3-4 minutes.

2. Add spinach leaves, salt, and pepper; stir fry for 1-2 minutes.
3. Add peas, crushed tomatoes, and chicken broth; simmer for 10-15 minutes on low flame.
4. Add to serving platter and top with parsley and lemon.
5. Serve and enjoy!

NUTRITION: Calories – 241 Fat –15 g Carbs – 19 g Protein – 9 g

91. Lentil Salad with Oranges

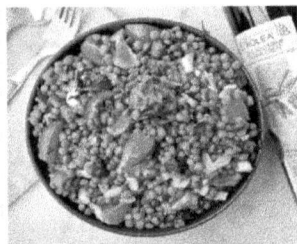

Preparation Time: 15 min.
Cooking Time: 0 min.
Serving: 2
INGREDIENTS:
- 0.4 lb. dry lentils, cooked
- 1 garlic clove, minced
- 0.3 lb. cherry tomatoes, diced
- 1 orange, peeled and cut into chunks
- ½ onion, diced
- 5-6 tablespoons fresh parsley, chopped
- 3 tablespoons extra virgin olive oil
- 2 tablespoons red wine vinegar
- Salt and pepper, as needed **DIRECTIONS:**

1. In a large mixing bowl add lentils, onion, tomatoes, parsley, and orange; mix thoroughly.
2. In a bowl add salt, pepper, garlic, olive oil, and red wine; stir to combine.
3. Drizzle dressing on salad. Toss well.
4. Serve and enjoy!

NUTRITION: Calories – 398 Fat –15 g Carbs – 47 g Protein – 17 g

92. Bell Peppers 'n Tomato-Chickpea Rice

Preparation time: 10 minutes
Cooking Time: 35 minutes
Serves: 4
INGREDIENTS:
- 2 tablespoons olive oil
- 1/2 chopped red bell pepper
- 1/2 chopped green bell pepper

- 1/2 chopped yellow pepper
- 1/2 chopped red pepper
- 1 medium onion, chopped
- 1 clove garlic, minced
- 2 cups cooked jasmine rice
- 1 teaspoon tomato paste
- 1 cup chickpeas
- salt to taste
- 1/2 teaspoon paprika
- 1 small tomato, chopped
- Parsley for garnish **DIRECTIONS:**

1. In a large mixing bowl, whisk well olive oil, garlic, tomato paste, and paprika. Season with salt generously.
2. Mix in rice and toss well to coat in the dressing.)add remaining ingredients and toss well to mix.)Let salad rest to allow flavors to mix for 15 minutes.) Toss one more time and adjust salt to taste if needed.
3. Garnish with parsley and serve.

NUTRITION: Calories: 490 Carbs: 93.0g Protein: 10.0g Fat: 8.0g

93. Seafood and Veggie Pasta

Preparation time: 5 minutes
Cooking time: 20 minutes
Serves: 4
INGREDIENTS:

- ¼ tsp. pepper
- ¼ tsp. salt
- 1 lb. raw shelled shrimp
- 1 lemon, cut into wedges
- 1 tbsp. butter
- 1 tbsp. olive oil
- 2 5-oz cans chopped clams, drained (reserve 2 tbsp. clam juice)
- 2 tbsp. dry white wine
- 4 cloves garlic, minced
- 4 cups zucchini, spiraled (use a veggie spiralizer)
- 4 tbsp. Parmesan Cheese
- Chopped fresh parsley to garnish **Directions:**

1. Ready the zucchini and spiral with a veggie paralyzer. Arrange 1 cup of zucchini noodle per bowl—a total of 4 bowls.
2. On medium fire, place a large nonstick saucepan and heat oil and butter.
3. For a minute, sauté garlic. Add shrimp and cook for 3 minutes until opaque or cooked.

4. Add white wine, reserved clam juice, and clams. Bring to a simmer and continue simmering for 2 minutes or until half of the liquid has evaporated. Stir constantly.
5. Season with pepper and salt. And if needed, add more to taste.
6. Remove from fire and evenly distribute seafood sauce to 4 bowls.
7. Top with a tablespoonful of Parmesan cheese per bowl, serve and enjoy.

NUTRITION: Calorie: 324.9 Carbs: 12g Protein: 43.8g Fat: 11.3g

94. Breakfast Salad from Grains and Fruits

Preparation time: 5 minutes
Cooking Time: 20 minutes
Serves: 6
INGREDIENTS:
- ¼ tsp. salt
- ¾ cup bulgur
- ¾ cup quick-cooking brown rice
- 1 8-oz low-fat vanilla yogurt
- 1 cup raisins
- 1 Granny Smith apple
- 1 orange
- 1 delicious red apple
- 3 cups water **DIRECTIONS:**

1. On high fire, place a large pot and bring water to a boil.
2. Add bulgur and rice. Lower fire to a simmer and cook for ten minutes while covered.
3. Turn off fire, set aside for 2 minutes while covered.
4. On a baking sheet, transfer and evenly spread grains to cool.
5. Meanwhile, peel oranges and cut them into sections. Chop and core apples.
6. Once grains are cool, transfer to a large serving bowl along with fruits.
7. Add yogurt and mix well to coat.
8. Serve and enjoy.

NUTRITION INFORMATION: Calorie: 48.6 Carbs: 23.9g Protein: 3.7g Fat: 1.1g

PIZZA

95. Funghi & Aglio Pizza

Preparation time: 5 minutes
Cooking Time: 20 minutes
Servings: 2
INGREDIENTS

- 1 cup flour
- ½ tsp. brown sugar
- 1 tsp. garlic powder
- 2 tsp. dried yeast
- ¼ tsp. salt
- 1 tbsp. olive oil
- 1 cup water
- 1 cup button mushrooms, chopped
- ¼ cup Gouda, grated
- 2 tbsp. tomato paste, sugar-free
- ½ tsp. dried oregano
- ¼ cup lukewarm water

DIRECTIONS

1. In a bowl fitted with a dough hook attachment, combine flour with brown sugar, dried yeast, and salt. Mix well and gradually add lukewarm water and oil. Continue to beat on high speed until smooth dough.
2. Transfer to a lightly floured surface and knead until entirely smooth. Form into a tight ball and wrap tightly in plastic foil. Set aside for one hour. Line a baking dish with some parchment paper and set it aside.
3. Roll out the dough with a rolling pin and transfer to the baking dish. Brush with tomato paste and sprinkle with oregano, Gouda, and button mushrooms. Add a trivet inside your Instant Pot and pour in 1 cup of water. Put the dish on the trivet. Seal the lid, and cook for 15 minutes on High Pressure. Do a quick release. Remove the pizza from the pot using a parchment paper. Cut and serve.

NUTRITION: Calories: 232 Fat: 11.8 Carb: 22.5 Protein: 2.8

96. Pizza Quattro Formaggi

Preparation time: 5 minutes
Cooking Time: 20 minutes
Servings: 4
INGREDIENTS

- 1 pizza crust
- ½ cup tomato paste
- ¼ cup water
- 1 tsp. dried oregano
- 1 oz. cheddar cheese
- 5-6 slices mozzarella
- ¼ cup grated gouda
- ¼ cup grated parmesan
- ½ cup grated gouda cheese
- 2 tbsp. extra virgin olive oil

DIRECTIONS

1. Grease the bottom of a baking dish with one tablespoon of olive oil. Line some parchment paper. Flour the working surface and roll out the pizza dough to the approximate size of your instant pot. Gently fit the dough in the previously prepared baking dish.
2. In a small bowl, combine tomato paste with water, and dry oregano. Spread the mixture over dough and finish with cheeses.
3. Add a trivet inside you're pot and pour in 1 cup of water. Seal the lid, and cook for 15 minutes on High Pressure. Do a quick release. Remove the pizza from the pot using parchment paper. Cut and serve.

NUTRITION: 250Cal 46%28gCarbs 37%10gFat 18%11gProtein

97. Turkey Pepperoni Pizza

Preparation time: 5 minutes
Cooking time: 20minutes
Servings: 4
INGREDIENTS

- 1 whole-wheat Italian pizza crust
- 1 cup fire-roasted tomatoes, diced
- 1 tsp. oregano
- ½ tsp. dried basil
- ½ cup turkey pepperoni, chopped
- 7 oz. Gouda cheese, grated
- 2 tbsp. olive oil

DIRECTIONS

1. Grease a baking pan with oil. Line some parchment paper and place the pizza crust in it.
2. Spread the fire-roasted tomatoes over the pizza crust and sprinkle with oregano and basil. Make a layer with cheese and top with pepperoni.
3. Add a trivet inside the pot and pour in 1 cup of water. Seal the lid, and cook for 15 minutes on High Pressure. Do a quick release. Remove the pizza from the pot using parchment paper.

NUTRITION: 210Cal 60%32gCarbs 21%5gFat 19%10gProtein

98. Tuna & Rosemary Pizza

Preparation time: 5 minutes
Cooking time: 25 minutes
Servings: 4
INGREDIENTS

- 1 cup canned tuna, oil-free
- ½ cup mozzarella cheese, shredded
- ¼ cup goat's cheese

- 3 tbsp. olive oil
- 1 tbsp. tomato paste
- ½ tsp. dried rosemary
- 14 oz. pizza crust
- 1 cup olives, optional

DIRECTIONS

1. Grease the bottom of a baking dish with one tablespoon of olive oil. Line some parchment paper. Flour the working surface and roll out the pizza dough to the approximate size of your instant pot. Gently fit the dough in the previously prepared baking dish.
2. In a bowl, combine olive oil, tomato paste, and rosemary. Whisk together and spread the mixture over the crust.
3. Sprinkle with goat cheese, mozzarella, and tuna. Place a trivet inside the pot and pour in 1 cup of water.
4. Seal the lid, and cook for 15 minutes on High Pressure. Do a quick release. Remove the pizza from the pot. Cut and serve.

NUTRITION: 153Cal 0%--Carbs 100%1gFat 0%--Protein

99. Tomato and Egg Breakfast Pizza

Preparation time: 5 minutes
Cooking time: 15 minutes
Serves 2
INGREDIENTS:
- 2 (6- to 8-inch-long) slices of whole-wheat nan bread
- 2 tablespoons prepared pesto
- 1 medium tomato, sliced
- 2 large eggs **DIRECTIONS:**

1. Heat a large nonstick skillet over medium-high heat. Place the naan bread in the skillet and let warm for about 2 minutes on each side, or until softened.
2. Spread 1 tablespoon of the pesto on one side of each slice and top with tomato slices.
3. Remove from the skillet and place each one on its plate.
4. Crack the eggs into the skillet, keeping them separated, and cook until the whites are no longer translucent and the yolk is cooked to desired doneness.
5. Using a spatula, spoon one egg onto each bread slice. Serve warm.

NUTRITION: Calories: 429 Fat: 16.8g Protein: 18.1g Carbs: 12.0g Fiber: 4.8g Sodium: 682mg

100. Easy Pizza Pockets

Preparation time: 10 minutes
Cooking time: 0 minutes
Serves 2

INGREDIENTS:

- ½ cup tomato sauce
- ½ teaspoon oregano
- ½ teaspoon garlic powder
- ½ cup chopped black olives
- 2 canned artichoke hearts, drained and chopped
- 2 ounces (57 g) pepperoni, chopped
- ½ cup shredded Mozzarella cheese
- 1 whole-wheat pita, halved **DIRECTIONS:**

1. In a medium bowl, stir together the tomato sauce, oregano, and garlic powder.
2. Add the olives, artichoke hearts, pepperoni, and cheese. Stir to mix.
3. Spoon the mixture into the pita halves and serve.

NUTRITION: Calories: 375 Fat: 23.5g Protein: 17.1g Carbs: 27.1g Fiber: 6.1g Sodium: 1080mg

101. Mushroom-Pesto Baked Pizza

Preparation time: 5 minutes
Cook time: 15 minutes
Serves 2
INGREDIENTS:

- 1 teaspoon extra-virgin olive oil
- ½ cup sliced mushrooms
- ½ red onion, sliced
- Salt and freshly ground black pepper
- ¼ cup store-bought pesto sauce
- 2 whole-wheat flatbreads
- ¼ cup shredded Mozzarella cheese **DIRECTIONS:**

1. Preheat the oven to 350ºF (180ºC).
2. In a small skillet, heat the oil over medium heat. Add the mushrooms and onion, and season with salt and pepper. Sauté for 3 to 5 minutes until the onion and mushrooms begin to soften.
3. Spread 2 tablespoons of pesto on each flatbread.
4. Divide the mushroom-onion mixture between the two flatbreads. Top each with 2 tablespoons of cheese.
5. Place the flatbreads on a baking sheet and bake for 10 to 12 minutes until the cheese is melted and bubbly. Serve warm.

NUTRITION: Calories: 348 Fat: 23.5g Protein: 14.2g Carbs: 28.1g Fiber: 7.1g Sodium: 792mg

SNACKS & DRINKS

102. Garlic and Tomato Bruschetta

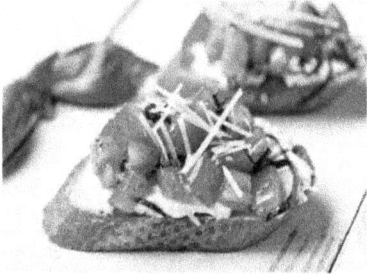

The flavor of garlic and the acidity of balsamic vinegar makes this snack one that you will have again and again. **Preparation Time:** 5 minutes
Cooking time: 5 minutes
Servings: 8
INGREDIENTS

- 8 slices ½-inch thick of a French baguette
- 1½ teaspoons minced fresh garlic
- 1¼ cups chopped plum tomatoes
- 1 teaspoon extra-virgin olive oil
- 1 teaspoon balsamic vinegar
- ½ teaspoon dried basil
- ¼ teaspoon of non-caloric sweetener
- ¼ teaspoon freshly ground pepper **DIRECTIONS:**

1. Preheat the oven to 500° F.
2. Take out a baking tray. Add olive oil to all sides of the baguette. Bake it for about 4 minutes.
3. Combine the remaining ingredients in a small bowl. Mix well.
4. Add the mixture to the baguette.

NUTRITION: Calories: 57 calories Protein: 2 g Total Fat: 1 g Carbohydrate: 11 g

103. Crostini

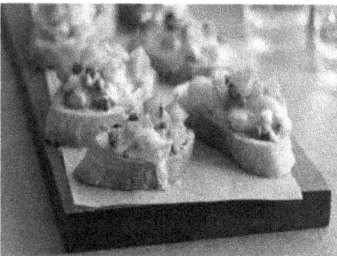

Another snack is featuring French baguette—this time, with the addition of herbs.
Preparation Time: 5 minutes
Cooking time: None
Servings: 25

INGREDIENTS

- 1 French baguette, roughly cut into ½-inch thick slices
- extra-virgin olive oil
- 2½ teaspoons fresh garlic paste
- minced fresh basil
- salt and freshly ground pepper to taste **DIRECTIONS:**

1. Preheat the oven to 375° F.
2. Take out a baking tray. Add olive oil to all sides of the baguette. Add garlic paste and pepper to taste, if you prefer. Bake it for about 4 minutes.
3. Top the baguette with basil, and enjoy!

NUTRITION: Calories: 41 calories Protein: 1 g Total Fat: 1 g Carbohydrate: 10 g

104. Baby Shrimps

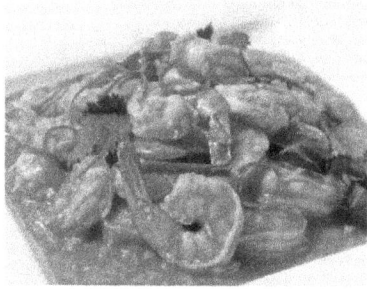

This snack is served on toasted rye and Dijon mustard, which enhances the dish's flavor profile.

Preparation Time: 5 minutes
Cooking time: 15 minutes
Servings: 12
INGREDIENTS

- ½ cup reduced-fat mayonnaise
- 1 tablespoon finely chopped fresh parsley
- 1 teaspoon Dijon mustard
- ½ teaspoon chopped capers
- 2 tablespoons finely minced shallot
- 1 bag cooked salad shrimp, thawed
- ¼ cup freshly squeezed lemon juice
- 16 paper-thin slices of lemon
- 16 pieces cocktail-sized, thin rye bread
- 2 tablespoons olive oil

DIRECTIONS:

1. Preheat the oven to 300° F.
2. In a small bowl, add parsley, mustard, mayonnaise, shallot, and capers. Mix them well and place them in the refrigerator for about an hour. Cover and refrigerate for no less than 1 hour to blend flavors.
3. Take a baking tray and place the rye slices. Coat them in olive oil and bake until they become crispy.
4. Add one teaspoon of mayonnaise on each rye toast. Top with 5 shrimps and sprinkle lemon juice on top. Top it with a slice of lemon.

NUTRITION: Calories: 47 calories Protein: 2 g Total Fat: 2 g Carbohydrate: 4 g

105. Spicy tomato to baked potatoes

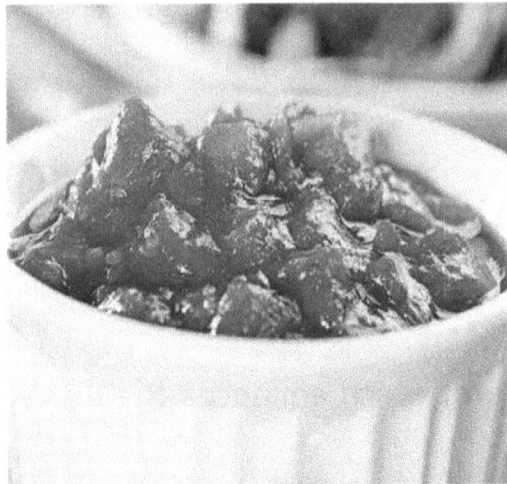

Serve with charcoal-baked or oven-baked potatoes.
Preparation Time: 5 minutes
Cooking time: 25 minutes
Servings: 4
INGREDIENTS

- ½ tbsp. Extra virgin olive oil
- 6 cloves
- Garlic
- 420g Canned tomatoes sliced
- ½ tsp. Paprika
- ½ tsp. Red Pepper flakes
- ¼ tsp. Salt **DIRECTIONS:**

1. Heat olive oil in a saucepan. Add chopped garlic and sauté for 1 minute.
2. Then add the tomatoes, paprika, red pepper flakes, and salt. Stir and cook for about 15–20 minutes, until the sauce is thickened to a ketchup state

NUTRITION: Calories: 59 calories Protein: 2 g Total Fat: 2.5 g Carbohydrate: 7.6 g

106. Green beans with warm dressing and bacon

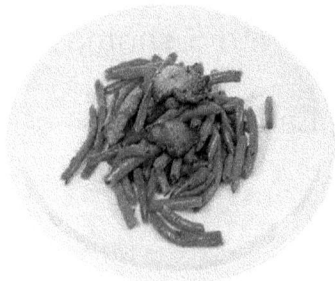

Servings: 2
Preparation Time: 5 minutes

Cooking time: 25 minutes
INGREDIENTS

- 2 pieces Bacon
- 1 Shallot
- 230g Green String Beans
- 2 tsp. White wine vinegar   **DIRECTIONS:**

1. Please, cook the beans, chopped into small pieces, in boiling salted water until soft, about 8 minutes. Drain and transfer to a bowl.
2. Meanwhile, sauté the chopped bacon in a well-heated skillet over medium heat until crisp. Put on a paper towel.
3. Put the finely chopped shallots into the pan and sauté for 30 seconds. Remove from heat and cool slightly. Add vinegar, salt, and pepper.
4. Pour beans with warm dressing and lay on top slices of bacon.

NUTRITION: Calories: 140 calories Protein: 7.3 g Total Fat: 9,2g Carbohydrate: 7.3 g

107. Rolls with lettuce

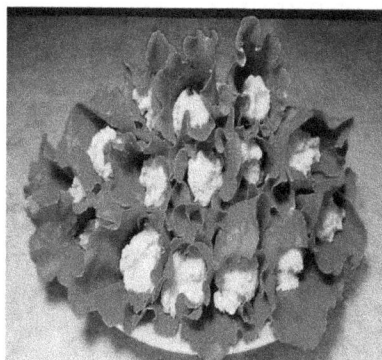

Preparation Time: 5 minutes
Cooking time: 15 minutes
Servings: 2
INGREDIENTS

- Green salad to taste
- 2 Egg
- 200g hard cheese
- 200g Peeled shrimp
- Low-calorie Mayonnaise to taste **DIRECTIONS:**

1. Prepare the filling for rolls—boil eggs and finely crush or grate. Grate the cheese. Finely chop the shrimp. Add some mayonnaise.
2. Put the cooked mass on lettuce leaves.
3. Gently wrap lettuce in rolls.

NUTRITION: Calories: 267 calories Protein: 25.2 g Total Fat: 17.2g Carbohydrate: 1.4 g

PASTA

108. Broccoli and Carrot Pasta Salad

Preparation time: 5 minutes
Cooking time: 10 minutes
Servings: 2
INGREDIENTS:

- 8 ounces (227 g) whole-wheat pasta
- 2 cups broccoli florets
- 1 cup peeled and shredded carrots
- ¼ cup plain Greek yogurt
- Juice of 1 lemon
- 1 teaspoon red pepper flakes
- Sea salt and freshly ground pepper, to taste **DIRECTIONS:**

1. Bring a large pot of lightly salted water to a boil. Add the pasta to the boiling water and cook until al dente. Drain and let rest for a few minutes.
2. When cooled, combine the pasta with the veggies, yogurt, lemon juice, and red pepper flakes in a large bowl, and stir thoroughly to combine.
3. Taste and season to taste with salt and pepper. Serve immediately.

NUTRITION: Calories: 428 Fat: 2.9g Protein: 15.9g Carbs: 84.6g Fiber: 11.7g Sodium: 642mg

109. Bean and Veggie Pasta

Preparation time: 10 minutes |
Cooking time: 15 minutes |
Servings: 2
INGREDIENTS:

- 16 ounces (454 g) small whole wheat pasta, such as penne, farfalle, or macaroni
- 5 cups water
- 1 (15-ounce / 425-g) can cannellini beans, drained and rinsed
- 1 (14.5-ounce / 411-g) can diced (with juice) or crushed tomatoes
- 1 yellow onion, chopped
- 1 red or yellow bell pepper, chopped
- 2 tablespoons tomato paste
- 1 tablespoon olive oil
- 3 garlic cloves, minced
- ¼ teaspoon crushed red pepper (optional)
- 1 bunch kale, stemmed and chopped
- 1 cup sliced basil

- ½ cup pitted Kalamata olives, chopped **DIRECTIONS:**
1. Add the pasta, water, beans, tomatoes (with juice if using diced), onion, bell pepper, tomato paste, oil, garlic, and crushed red pepper (if desired), to a large stockpot or deep skillet with a lid. Bring to a boil over high heat, stirring often.
2. Reduce the heat to medium-high, add the kale, and cook, continuing to stir often, until the pasta is al dente, about 10 minutes.
3. Remove from the heat and let sit for 5 minutes. Garnish with the basil and olives and serve.

NUTRITION: Calories: 565 Fat: 17.7g Protein: 18.0g Carbs: 85.5g Fiber: 16.5g

Sodium: 540mg

110. Roasted Ratatouille Pasta

Preparation time: 10 minutes
Cooking time: 30 minutes
Servings: 2
INGREDIENTS:
- 1 small eggplant (about 8 ounces / 227 g)
- 1 small zucchini
- 1 portobello mushroom
- 1 Roma tomato, halved

- ½ medium sweet red pepper, seeded
- ½ teaspoon salt, plus additional for the pasta water
- 1 teaspoon Italian herb seasoning
- 1 tablespoon olive oil
- 2 cups farfalle pasta (about 8 ounces / 227 g)
- 2 tablespoons minced sun-dried tomatoes in olive oil with herbs
- 2 tablespoons prepared pesto **DIRECTIONS:**

1. Slice the ends off the eggplant and zucchini. Cut them lengthwise into ½-inch slices.
2. Place the eggplant, zucchini, mushroom, tomato, and red pepper in a large bowl and sprinkle with ½ teaspoon of salt. Using your hands, toss the vegetables well so that they're covered evenly with the salt. Let them rest for about 10 minutes.
3. While the vegetables are resting, preheat the oven to 400ºF (205ºC). Line a baking sheet with parchment paper.
4. When the oven is hot, drain off any liquid from the vegetables and pat them dry with a paper towel. Add the Italian herb seasoning and olive oil to the vegetables and toss well to coat both sides.
5. Lay the vegetables out in a single layer on the baking sheet. Roast them for 15 to 20 minutes, flipping them over after about 10 minutes or once they start to brown on the underside. When the vegetables are charred in spots, remove them from the oven.
6. While the vegetables are roasting, fill a large saucepan with water. Add salt and cook the pasta until al dente, about 8 to 10 minutes. Drain the pasta, reserving ½ cup of the pasta water.
7. When cool enough to handle, cut the vegetables into large chunks (about 2 inches) and add them to the hot pasta.
8. Stir in the sun-dried tomatoes and pesto and toss everything well. Serve immediately.

NUTRITION: Calories: 613 Fat: 16.0g Protein: 23.1g Carbs: 108.5g Fiber: 23.0g Sodium: 775mg

111. Lentil and Mushroom Pasta

Preparation time: 10 minutes
Cooking time: 50 minutes
Serves 2
INGREDIENTS:
- 2 tablespoons olive oil
- 1 large yellow onion, finely diced
- 2 portobello mushrooms, trimmed and chopped finely
- 2 tablespoons tomato paste
- 3 garlic cloves, chopped
- 1 teaspoon oregano

- 2½ cups water
- 1 cup brown lentils
- 1 (28-ounce / 794-g) can diced tomatoes with basil (with juice if diced)
- 1 tablespoon balsamic vinegar
- 8 ounces (227 g) pasta of choice, cooked
- Salt and black pepper, to taste
- Chopped basil, for garnish **DIRECTIONS:**

1. Place a large stockpot over medium heat. Add the oil. Once the oil is hot, add the onion and mushrooms. Cover and cook until both are soft, about 5 minutes. Add the tomato paste, garlic, and oregano and cook 2 minutes, stirring constantly.
2. Stir in the water and lentils. Bring to a boil, then reduce the heat to mediumlow and cook for 5 minutes, covered.
3. Add the tomatoes (and juice if using diced) and vinegar. Replace the lid, reduce the heat to low and cook until the lentils are tender, about 30 minutes.
4. Remove the sauce from the heat and season with salt and pepper to taste. Garnish with the basil and serve over the cooked pasta.

NUTRITION: Calories: 463 Fat: 15.9g Protein: 12.5g Carbs: 70.8g Fiber: 16.9g Sodium: 155mg

112. Tomato Basil Pasta

Preparation time: 3 minutes
Cooking time: 2 minutes
Serves 2
INGREDIENTS:
- 2 cups dried campanelle or similar pasta

- 1¾ cups vegetable stock
- ½ teaspoon salt, plus more as needed
- 2 tomatoes, cut into large dices
- 1 or 2 pinches red pepper flakes
- ½ teaspoon garlic powder
- ½ teaspoon dried oregano
- 10 to 12 fresh sweet basil leaves
- Freshly ground black pepper, to taste **DIRECTIONS:**

1. In your Instant Pot, stir together the pasta, stock, and salt. Scatter the tomatoes on top (do not stir).
2. Secure the lid. Select the Manual mode and set the cooking time for 2 minutes at High Pressure.
3. Once cooking is complete, do a quick pressure release? Carefully open the lid.
4. Stir in the red pepper flakes, oregano, and garlic powder. If there's more than a few tablespoons of liquid in the bottom, select Sauté and cook for 2 to 3 minutes until it evaporates.
5. When ready to serve, chiffonade the basil and stir it in. Taste and season with more salt and pepper, as needed. Serve warm.

NUTRITION: Calories: 415 Fat: 2.0g Protein: 15.2g Carbs: 84.2g Fiber: 5.0g Sodium: 485mg

DESSERT

113. Almond and Chocolate Butter Dip

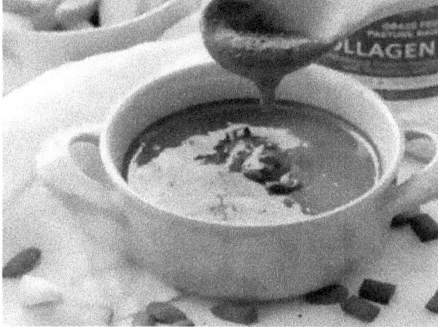

Preparation Time: 15 minutes
Cooking Time: 10 minute
Serving: 14
INGREDIENTS

- 1 cup Plain Greek Yogurt
- ½ cup almond butter
- 1/3 cup chocolate hazelnut spread
- 1 tablespoon honey
- 1 teaspoon vanilla
- Sliced fruits such as pears, apples, apricots, bananas, etc.

DIRECTIONS:

1. Take a medium-sized bowl and add the first five listed ingredients.
2. With an immersion blender, blend well until you have a smooth dip.
3. Serve with your favorite sliced fruit.
4. Enjoy!

NUTRITION: Calories: 115 Fat: 8g Carbohydrates: 115g Protein: 4g

114. Strawberry and Feta Delight

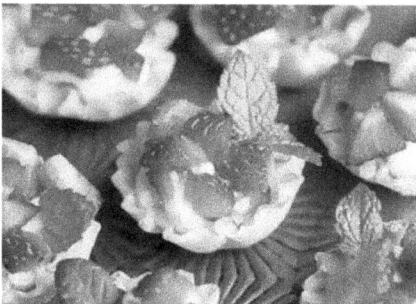

Preparation time: 10 minutes
Cooking Time: 0
Serving: 4
INGREDIENTS

- 4 cups baby spinach
- 6 ounces feta cheese, crumbled
- 1 cup fresh strawberries, thinly sliced
- ½ cup walnuts, chopped
- Balsamic Dijon vinaigrette
- 2 tablespoons extra-virgin olive oil
- 2 tablespoons balsamic vinegar
- 1 tablespoon Dijon mustard
- 1 tablespoon honey
- Salt and pepper as needed **DIRECTIONS:**

1. Take a small-sized glass bowl and mix in the olive oil, Dijon mustard, balsamic vinegar, and honey.
2. Season with some pepper and salt.
3. Add the spinach, strawberries, feta, walnuts, and pine nuts to a large-sized mixing bowl.
4. Divide the mixture amongst serving plates and dress with the previously prepared vinaigrette dressing.
5. Serve

NUTRITION: Calories: 270 Fat: 22g Carbohydrates: 11g Protein: 9g

115. Simple Strawberry Yogurt Ice Cream

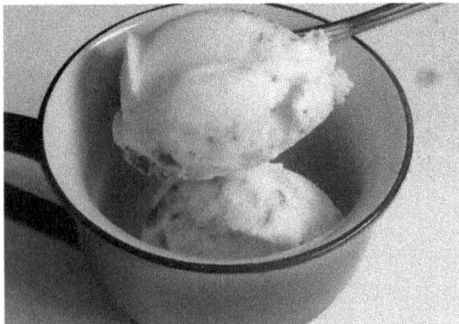

Preparation Time: 10 minutes
Cooking Time: 20 minutes
Serving: 4
INGREDIENTS
- 3 cups of plain Greek low-fat yogurt
- 1 cup of sugar
- ¼ cup of freshly squeezed lemon juice
- 2 teaspoons of vanilla
- 1/8 teaspoon of salt
- 1 cup of sliced strawberries

DIRECTIONS:
1. Take a medium-sized bowl and add yogurt, lemon juice, and sugar, vanilla, and salt.

2. Whisk the whole mixture well.
3. Freeze the yogurt mix into a 2-quart ice cream maker according to the given instructions.
4. Make sure to add sliced strawberries during the final minute.
5. Transfer the yogurt to an airtight container.
6. Freeze for another 2-4 hours.
7. Allow standing for about 5-15 minutes.
8. Serve and enjoy!

NUTRITION: Calories: 86 Fat: 1g Carbohydrates: 16g Protein: 4g

116. Pear with Honey Drizzles

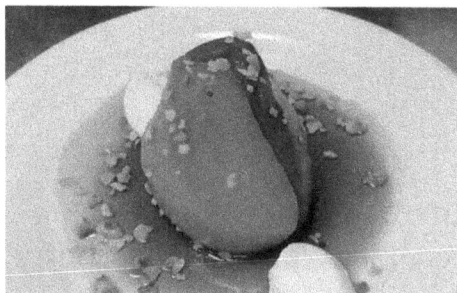

Preparation Time: 10 minutes
Cooking Time: 20 minutes
Serving: 4
INGREDIENTS

- 3 pieces of ripe medium Bosc of Bartlett pears. Peel and core, then slice into halves
- ¼ cup of pear nectar
- 3 tablespoons of honey
- 2 tablespoons of butter
- 1 teaspoon of orange zest
- ½ cup of mascarpone cheese
- 2 tablespoons of powdered sugar
- 1/3 cup of chopped up roasted salted pistachio **DIRECTIONS:**
1. Preheat your oven to 400 degrees Fahrenheit.
2. Take a baking dish and add pears, making sure to arrange them with the cut side facing down.
3. Add the next four listed ingredients.
4. Roast for 20-25 minutes until tender.
5. Transfer the pears to a serving dish and pour the cooking liquid on top.
6. Take a bowl and stir in mascarpone cheese and powdered sugar.
7. Spoon the mix over the pears.
8. Sprinkle with pistachio and drizzle honey.
9. Enjoy!

NUTRITION: Calories: 250 Fat: 8g Carbohydrates: 27g Protein: 3g

117. Cherry and Olive Bites

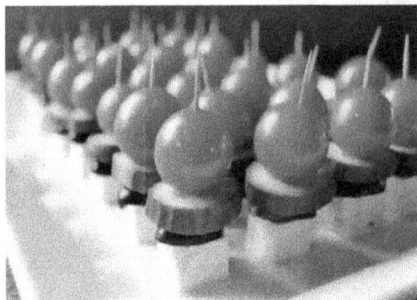

Preparation time: 15 minutes
Cook Time: 0
Serving: 30
INGREDIENTS

- 24 cherry tomatoes, halved
- 24 black olives, pitted
- 24 feta cheese cubes
- 24 toothpick/decorative skewers **DIRECTIONS:**

1. Use a toothpick or skewer and thread feta cheese, black olives, and cherry tomato halves in that order.
2. Repeat until all the ingredients are use.
3. Arrange in a serving platter.
4. Serve and enjoy!

NUTRITION: Calories: 57 Fat: 5g Carbohydrates: 2g Protein: 2g

118. Fluffed Up Chocolate Mousse

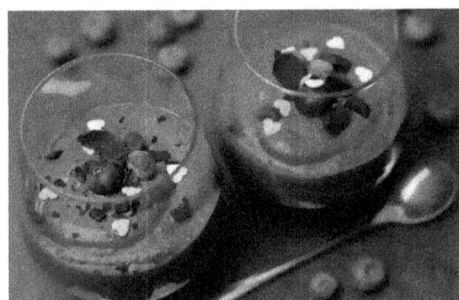

Preparation Time: 5 minutes
Cook Time: 0
Serving: 4
INGREDIENTS

- 1 can (14.5 ounces) coconut cream, chilled
- 3 tablespoons unsweetened cocoa powder
- ¼ cup Swerve
- 1 teaspoon vanilla extract **DIRECTIONS:**

1. Take a large-sized mixing bowl and add coconut cream, whip with a hand mixer.

2. Keep whipping for 3 minutes until fluffy.
3. Fold in cocoa powder, vanilla, swerve and mix.
4. Serve immediately!

NUTRITION: Calories: 222 Fat: 22g Carbohydrates: 4g Protein: 1g

119. Chocolate Butter Dip

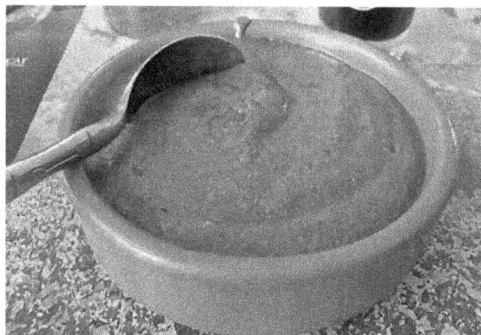

Preparation Time: 15 minutes
Cooking Time: 0 minutes
Serving: 14
INGREDIENTS

- 1 cup of Plain Greek Yogurt
- ½ cup of almond butter
- 1/3 cup of chocolate hazelnut spread
- 1 tablespoon of honey
- 1 teaspoon of vanilla
- Sliced up fruits as desired, such as pears, apples, apricots, bananas, etc.

DIRECTIONS:

1. Take a medium-sized bowl and add the first five listed ingredients.
2. With an immersion blender, blend well until you have a smooth dip.
3. Serve with your favorite sliced fruit.
4. Enjoy!

NUTRITION: Calories: 115 Fat: 8g Carbohydrates: 115g Protein: 4g

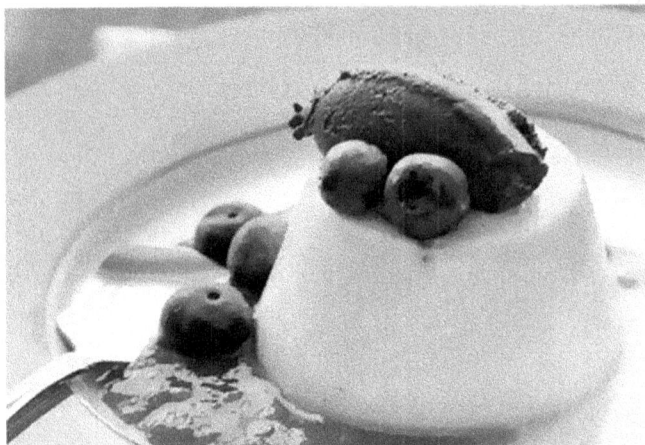

Preparation Time: 5 minutes
Cooking Time: 10 minutes
Serving: 4
INGREDIENTS

- 2 cups of freshly divided mixed berries
- 1 package of plain gelatin powder
- 1 cup of milk
- 1 2/3 cup of heavy cream
- ¾ cup of divided sugar **DIRECTIONS:**

1. Place 1 cup of raspberries into a food processor.
2. Process it to turn into a puree.
3. Take a small saucepan and transfer the puree to that saucepan.
4. Add about ¼ cup of sugar and the remaining raspberries.
5. Cook over medium heat for 10 minutes, making sure to stir from time to time.
6. Remove the heat after 10 minutes and let cool.
7. Cover and chill in your fridge.
8. Take another saucepan and combine your milk and gelatin and wait until the gelatin softens.
9. Simmer over medium heat and keep frequently stirring to dissolve the gelatin fully.
10. Stir heavy cream alongside the rest of the sugar and cook for another 3-5 minutes until the sugar is mixed.
11. Pour the mixture into 4 ramekins.
12. Chill them for 8 hours or overnight.
13. Invert the mold and place it on a serving plate.
14. Once the Panna Cotta comes out, top it with your berry compote.
15. Serve.

NUTRITION: Calories: 191 Fat: 15g Carbohydrates: 6g Protein: 9g

28 DAY MEAL PLAN

DAYS	BREAKFAST	LUNCH	DINNER
1	Eggs with Zucchini Noodles	Grilled Sardines & Arugula	Mussels with tomatoes & chili
2	Avocado and Apple Smoothie	Tuna Pasta with Artichokes	Thai Tuna Bowl
3	Avocado Toast	Greek Salmon Burgers	Baked Cod in Parchment
4	Berry Oats	Fruity Chicken Salad	
5	Mini Frittatas	Garlic Broiled Sardines	Chicken Gyros with Tzatziki
6	Quinoa and Eggs Pan	Tomato & Pasta Bowl	Chicken with Onions, Potatoes, Figs, and Carrots
7	Stuffed Tomatoes	Cheese Stuffed Tomatoes	Rosemary Baked Chicken Drumsticks
8	Eggs with Zucchini Noodles	Easy Chicken Greek Salad	One-Pan Tuscan Chicken
9	Avocado and Apple Smoothie	Grilled Sardines & Arugula	Bell Peppers on Chicken Breasts
10	Sun-dried Tomatoes Oatmeal	Flank Steak & Spinach Salad	Beef Brisket and Veggies
11	Scrambled Eggs	Chicken & Garbanzo Salad	Stewed Chicken Greek Style
12	Lentil Salmon Salad	Greek Chicken Stew	Greek Salmon Burgers
13	Garlic Caper Beef Roast	Salmon Panzanella	Pita Chicken Burger with Spicy Yogurt
14	Yummy Turkey Meatballs	Mediterranean Tuna Salad	Meatloaf
15	Roasted Fish & New Potatoes	Grilled Sardines & Arugula	Turkey Burgers with Mango Salsa
16	Chicken Sausage and Peppers	Seafood Couscous Paella	Pork Chops and Herbed Tomato Sauce

17	Mozzarella and Pears Salad	Bulgur Salad	Steak with Red Wine–Mushroom Sauce
18	Avocado and Apple Smoothie	Greek Salmon Burgers	Greek Meatballs (Keftedes)
19	Zucchini in Greek	Easy Chicken Greek Salad	Mozzarella and Pears Salad
20	Watermelon "Pizza"	Tasty Lamb Ribs	Peppers and Lentils Salad
21	Avocado Toast		Spicy Shrimp Salad
22	Sun-dried Tomatoes Oatmeal	Greek Chicken Stew	Pepper Tilapia with Spinach
23	Peas and Ham Thick Soup	Mediterranean Tuna Salad	Sweet and Sour Spinach Salad
24	Eggs with Zucchini Noodles	Chicken & Garbanzo Salad	Pita Chicken Burger with Spicy Yogurt
25	Avocado and Apple Smoothie	Flank Steak & Spinach Salad	Pork Chops and Herbed Tomato Sauce
26	Scalloped Tomatoes	Salmon Panzanella	Meatloaf
27	Olives and Lentils Salad	Tuna Pasta with Artichokes	Beef and Zucchini Skillet
28	Berry Oats	Seafood Couscous Paella	Hot Pork Meatballs

CONCLUSION

Overall, the Mediterranean diet is a healthy way to eat. On eating whole foods like fruits, vegetables, grains, legumes, and nuts. It's low in saturated fats and calories while also being high in fiber, vitamins, and minerals. The Mediterranean diet is one of the world's healthiest diets. It teaches people how to eat in a way that's good for their body and their brain. The Mediterranean diet's key is eating a diet rich in fruits, vegetables, and whole grains.

The diet consists of fruits, vegetables, legumes, grains, dairy products, and fish. The Complete Mediterranean Diet Cookbook is an excellent book for women who want to eat healthily and lose weight. If you're looking for a cookbook that's full of easy to follow recipes, this is the book for you. The Complete Mediterranean Diet Cookbook includes over 200 delicious recipes that are certified by the Mediterranean Diet Foundation. It's not just full of fresh produce, and it's also low in dairy and meats. If you want to eat a healthy diet, you need to pay attention to the Mediterranean Diet. The Mediterranean Diet has to be effective in preventing heart disease. If you follow the Mediterranean diet, you will not only have a healthy and balanced lifestyle, but your skin will also improve.

Many different diets will work for you, but the Mediterranean diet is a great place to start. It combines all the best health practices into one diet: fruits, vegetables, whole grains, and beans. The Complete Mediterranean Diet Cookbook is a musthave cookbook for anyone interested in a healthy diet.

The Complete Mediterranean Diet's goal is to help you achieve optimal health with a balanced diet that includes all the food groups and essential nutrients. The Complete Mediterranean Diet Cookbook is a spectacular book that explains the health benefits of eating like a Greek. It's an excellent book for cooking enthusiasts and people who want to eat healthier and live longer. The Mediterranean Diet is a diet that has been around for thousands of years. It's known for its focus on fruits, vegetables, fish, and whole grains. The benefits of the Mediterranean diet are numerous.

The Mediterranean Diet is a great plan to follow for those looking to lose weight, be healthy, and live longer. The Mediterranean diet is low in calories and rich in health benefits. The best way to cook and eat healthily is to follow the Mediterranean Diet. This diet encourages eating lots of fresh fruit, vegetables, and whole grains. The Mediterranean Diet is one of the most famous and influential diets globally, but this new cookbook covers all the bases for a healthy diet. The Complete Mediterranean Diet is a healthy diet that combines what the Mediterranean Diet is all about. The Complete Mediterranean Diet's goal is to help you achieve optimal health with a balanced diet that includes all the food groups and essential nutrients. The Complete Mediterranean Diet Cookbook is a spectacular book that explains the health benefits of eating like a Greek. It's an excellent book for cooking enthusiasts and people who want to eat healthier and live longer. The Mediterranean Diet is a diet that has been around for thousands of years. It's known for its focus on fruits, vegetables, fish, and whole grains. The benefits of the Mediterranean diet are numerous.

www.ingramcontent.com/pod-product-compliance
Lightning Source LLC
Chambersburg PA
CBHW080627030426
42336CB00018B/3100

9 781803 613727